Communications in Computer and Information Science 578

Commenced Publication in 2007
Founding and Former Series Editors:
Alfredo Cuzzocrea, Dominik Ślęzak, and Xiaokang Yang

More information about this series at http://www.springer.com/series/7899

Markus Helfert · Andreas Holzinger
Martina Ziefle · Ana Fred
John O'Donoghue · Carsten Röcker (Eds.)

Information and Communication Technologies for Ageing Well and e-Health

First International Conference, ICT4AgeingWell 2015
Lisbon, Portugal, May 20–22, 2015
Revised Selected Papers

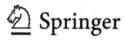 Springer

Editors

Markus Helfert
School of Computing
Dublin City University
Dublin
Ireland

Andreas Holzinger
Human-Computer Interaction
Medical University of Graz
Graz
Austria

Martina Ziefle
RWTH Aachen University
Aachen
Germany

Ana Fred
Instituto Superior Técnico, Instituto de
 Telecomunicações
Technical University of Lisbon
Lisboa
Portugal

John O'Donoghue
Imperial College London
London
UK

Carsten Röcker
System Technology and Image Exploitation
Fraunhofer Institute of Optonics
Lemgo
Germany

ISSN 1865-0929   ISSN 1865-0937 (electronic)
Communications in Computer and Information Science
ISBN 978-3-319-27694-6   ISBN 978-3-319-27695-3 (eBook)
DOI 10.1007/978-3-319-27695-3

Library of Congress Control Number: 2015956371

This Springer imprint is published by SpringerNature
The registered company is Springer International Publishing AG Switzerland

Preface

This book includes extended and revised versions of a set of selected papers from ICT4AgeingWell 2015 (The International Conference on Information and Communication Technologies for Ageing Well and e-Health), held in Lisbon, Portugal, May 20–22, 2015, which was sponsored by the Institute for Systems and Technologies of Information, Control and Communication (INSTICC) and held in cooperation with the International Society for Telemedicine & eHealth - ISfTeH, European Health Telematics Association – EHTEL, and the AAL Programme.

The purpose of the ICT4AgeingWell series of conferences is to bring together researchers and practitioners interested in methodologies and applications related to the field of information and communication technologies for ageing well and e-health. It has five main topic areas, covering different aspects, including ambient-assisted living, telemedicine and e-health, monitoring, accessibility and user interfaces, robotics and devices for independent living, and HCI for ageing populations.

The program of this conference included several outstanding keynote lectures presented by internationally renowned distinguished researchers who are experts in the various ICT4AgeingWell areas, including (alphabetically): Juan Carlos Augusto (School of Science and Technology, Middlesex University, UK), Thomas Hermann (CITEC - Center of Excellence Cognitive Interaction Technology, Bielefeld University, Germany), Victor Chang (Leeds Beckett University, UK), and William Molloy (Centre for Gerontology and Rehabilitation, School of Medicine, UCC, Ireland). Their keynote speeches heightened the overall quality of the program and significance of the theme of the conference.

We received 45 paper submissions from 28 countries in all continents, of which 27 % were accepted as full papers. The high quality of the papers received imposed difficult choices in the review process. Each submission was evaluated via, a double-blind review process by the Program Committee, whose members are highly qualified independent researchers in the ICT4AgeingWell 2015 topic areas.

This book contains the revised papers selected among the best contributions taking also into account the quality of their presentation at the conference, as assessed by the session chairs. We hope you find these papers interesting, and we trust they will represent a helpful reference for all those who need to address any of the aforementioned research areas.

We wish to thank all those who supported and helped to organize the conference. On behalf of the conference Organizing Committee, we would like to thank the authors, whose work mostly contributed to a very successful conference, and to the members of the Program Committee, whose expertise and diligence were instrumental for the quality of the final contributions. We also wish to thank all the members of the

Organizing Committee, whose work and commitment were invaluable. Last but not least, we would like to thank Springer for their collaboration in getting this book to print.

September 2015

Ana Fred
Andreas Holzinger
Carsten Röcker
John O'Donoghue
Markus Helfert
Martina Ziefle

Organization

Conference Co-chairs

Markus Helfert   Dublin City University, Ireland
Andreas Holzinger   Medical University Graz, Austria

Program Co-chairs

Martina Ziefle   RWTH-Aachen University, Germany
Ana Fred   Instituto de Telecomunicações/IST, Portugal
John O'Donoghue   Imperial College London, UK
Carsten Röcker   Ostfestfalen-Lippe UAS and Fraunhofer IOSB-INA, Germany

Program Committee

Marco Aiello   University of Groningen, The Netherlands
Dietrich Albert   University of Graz and Graz University of Technology, Austria
Carlo Alberto Avizzano   Scuola Superiore Sant'Anna, Italy
Angel Barriga   IMSE-CNM-CSIC, Spain
Karsten Berns   Robotics Research Lab, Germany
Frada Burstein   Faculty of IT, Monash University, Australia
Stuart Cunningham   Glyndwr University, UK
Mary Czerwinski   Microsoft Research, USA
Maria Luisa Damiani   Università degli Studi di Milano, Italy
Monica Divitini   Norwegian University of Science and Technology, Norway
Deborah I. Fels   Ryerson University, Canada
Jinjuan Heidi Feng   Towson University (Baltimore Hebrew University), USA
Ana Fred   Instituto de Telecomunicações/IST, Portugal
Diamantino Freitas   Faculdade de Engenharia da Universidade do Porto, Portugal
Ennio Gambi   Università Politecnica Delle Marche, Italy
Todor Ganchev   Technical University of Varna, Bulgaria
Jaakko Hakulinen   University of Tampere, Finland
Dirk Heylen   Human Media Interaction, University of Twente, The Netherlands
Alina Huldtgren   Eindhoven University of Technology, Germany
Kyoung-Don Kang   Binghamton University, USA
David Kaufman   Simon Fraser University, Canada

Takahiro Kawamura	Toshiba Corp., Japan
Peter Kokol	University of Maribor, Slovenia
Herman van der Kooij	University of Twente, The Netherlands
Andrej Kos	University of Ljubljana, Slovenia
Mikel Larrea	Universidad del País Vasco, Spain
Barbara Leporini	ISTI - CNR, Italy
Christine Lisetti	Florida International University, USA
Linda Little	Northumbria University, UK
Thurmon Lockhart	Arizona State University, USA
Piero Malcovati	University of Pavia, Italy
Roberto Manduchi	University of California Santa Cruz, USA
Kathleen F. McCoy	University of Delaware, USA
Nirvana Meratnia	University of Twente, The Netherlands
Hiroshi Mineno	Shizuoka University, Japan
Elena Mugellini	University of Applied Sciences Western Switzerland, Switzerland
Majid Nabi	Eindhoven University of Technology, The Netherlands
Keiichi Nakata	University of Reading, UK
Amit Anil Nanavati	IBM Research, India
Lorenzo Natale	Istituto Italiano di Tecnologia, Italy
Anthony F. Norcio	UMBC (University of Maryland Baltimore County), USA
Masayuki Numao	Osaka University, Japan
Angelo Oddi	Consiglio Nazionale delle Ricerche, Italy
John O'Donoghue	Imperial College London, UK
Patrizio Pelliccione	University of Gothenburg, Sweden
Ronald H. Perrott	Oxford e-Research Centre, UK
Niels Pinkwart	Humboldt University, Germany
Ronald Poppe	Utrecht University, The Netherlands
Marco Porta	Università degli Studi di Pavia, Italy
Girijesh Prasad	University of Ulster, UK
Klaus Radermacher	RWTH Aachen University, Germany
Bernd Radig	Technische Universität München, Germany
Gregorio Robles	Universidad Rey Juan Carlos, Spain
Wendy Rogers	Georgia Institute of Technology, USA
Philippe Roose	LIUPPA/IUT de Bayonne/UPPA, France
Corina Sas	Lancaster University, UK
Sreela Sasi	Gannon University, USA
Fabio A. Schreiber	Politecnico di Milano, Italy
Loren Schwiebert	Wayne State University, USA
Bryan W. Scotney	University of Ulster, UK
Yuzhong Shen	Old Dominion University, USA
Josep Silva	Universidad Politécnica de Valencia, Spain
Luca Spalazzi	Università Politecnica Delle Marche, Italy
Christine Strauss	University of Vienna, Austria
Frans R.J. Verhey	Maastricht University, The Netherlands
Salvatore Vitabile	Università degli Studi di Palermo, Italy

Gerhard Weber   Technical University of Dresden, Germany
Martin White   University of Sussex, UK
George Xylomenos   Athens University of Economics and Business, Greece
Xenophon Zabulis   Foundation for Research and Technology Hellas
                       (FORTH), Greece

Additional Reviewer

Lucia Pepa   DII, Dipartimento di Ingegneria dell'Informazione
                       (UNIVPM), Italy

Invited Speakers

Juan Carlos Augusto   School of Science and Technology,
                       Middlesex University, UK
Victor Chang   Leeds Beckett University, UK
Thomas Hermann   CITEC - Center of Excellence Cognitive Interaction
                       Technology, Bielefeld University, Germany
William Molloy   Centre for Gerontology and Rehabilitation,
                       School of Medicine, UCC, Ireland

Contents

Monitoring, Accessibility and User Interfaces

HCI for Ageing Populations

Invited Papers

The Community Assessment of Risk and Treatment Strategies (CARTS): An Integrated Care Pathway to Manage Frailty and Functional Decline in Community Dwelling Older Adults

Rónán O' Caoimh[1,2,12(✉)], Elizabeth Weathers[1,3(✉)], Ruth Hally[1],
Ronan O' Sullivan[1], Carol FitzGerald[1], Nicola Cornally[1,3],
Anton Svendrovski[4], Elizabeth Healy[5], Elizabeth O'Connell[6],
Gabrielle O'Keeffe[7], Patricia Leahy Warren[3], Brian D. Daly[1],
Roger Clarnette[8], Suzanne Smith[9], Niamh Cipriani[9], Rodd Bond[9,12],
Francesc Orfila[10], Constança Paúl[11], and D. William Molloy[1,12]

[1] Centre for Gerontology and Rehabilitation, College of Medicine and Health, University College Cork, Cork City, Ireland
rocaoimh@hotmail.com, {e.weathers, ruth.hally, r.osullivan, carol.fitzgerald, n.cornally, w.molloy}@ucc.ie, briandaly84@gmail.com

[2] Health Research Board Clinical Research Facility Galway, National University of Ireland, Galway, Geata an Eolais, University Road, Galway, Ireland

[3] School of Nursing and Midwifery, University College Cork, Cork City, Ireland
{e.weathers, n.cornally, Patricia.Leahy}@ucc.ie

[4] UZIK Consulting Inc., 86 Gerrard St E, Unit 12D, Toronto, ON M5B 2J1, Canada
info@statshelp.ca

[5] Centre for Public Health Nursing, Ballincollig and Bishopstown, Co Cork, Ireland
elizabeth.healy@hse.ie

[6] Centre for Public Health Nursing, Mahon and Ballintemple, Cork City, Ireland
elizabeth.oconnell@hse.ie

[7] Health Service Executive, South Lee, Cork, Ireland
gabrielle.okeeffe@hse.ie

[8] School of Medicine and Pharmacology, University of Western Australia, Crawley, Australia
roger.clarnette@health.wa.gov.au

[9] Netwell Centre and Louth Age Friendly County Initiative, Co Louth, Ireland
{Suzanne.smith, Rodd.bond}@netwellcentre.org, niamh.caprani@casala.ie

[10] Institute for Research Primary Healthcare, Jordi Gol University, Barcelona, Spain
forfila.bcn.ics@gencat.cat

[11] Institute of Biomedical Sciences Abel Salazar, University of Porto, Porto, Portugal
constancapaul@gmail.com

[12] COLLAGE (COLLaboration on AGEing), University College Cork, Cork City and Louth Age Friendly County Initiative, Co Louth, Ireland

M. Helfert et al. (Eds.): ICT4AgeingWell 2015, CCIS 578, pp. 3–18, 2015.
DOI: 10.1007/978-3-319-27695-3_1

Abstract. The Community Assessment of Risk & Treatment Strategies (CARTS) is an evolving integrated care pathway for community-dwelling older adults, designed to screen for and prevent frailty through the use of innovative, novel targeted risk screening instruments, comprehensive geriatric assessment, tailored interventions and integrated patient-centred multi-disciplinary monitoring. This multimodal service aims to positively affect risk and frailty transitions, to reduce adverse healthcare outcomes and achieve the European Innovation Partnerships on Active and Healthy Ageing's (EIP-AHA) goal of improved healthy life years. The CARTS programme builds on the activities and deliverables defined within Action Plan A3 of the EIP-AHA 'Prevention and early diagnosis of frailty, both physical and cognitive, in older people', aiming to use information and communications technology (ICT) to facilitate its implementation in clinical practice. The CARTS instruments have been piloted in Ireland as well as in Portugal, Spain and Australia. An update on the research conducted to date and future plans are presented.

Keywords: Frailty · Community-Screening · Assessment · Risk · Integrated care pathways

1 Introduction

Population ageing is occurring throughout the European Union (EU) [1] and is associated with an increased prevalence of frailty [2], disability and chronic medical comorbidities [3]. While frailty is often found in those with comorbidity and disability, it is recognised as a distinct clinical condition. Frailty is a multi-factorial, age-associated decline in the ability to manage stressors and commonly occurs in vulnerable older adults [4]. Estimates of frailty vary, with a recent systematic review suggesting an overall weighted prevalence of 10.7 % in those aged over 65 years [5]. Frailty is associated with the risk of developing adverse healthcare outcomes including institutionalisation [6], hospitalisation [7] and death [8, 9]. Frailty also negatively affects patient quality of life [10] and increases healthcare costs [11, 12]. Although associated with ageing, it is not an inevitable part of the ageing process. Frailty is suggested to be reversible, particularly when it is independent of disease and disability [13, 14]. If identified at its earliest stage, the pre-frail state, it may be prevented. Given the ageing population, there is a need to develop suitable strategies to reverse or prevent frailty and thereby prevent functional decline, impairment in activities of daily living (ADL) and consequent disability.

Comprehensive geriatric assessment (CGA) describes a broad interdisciplinary assessment to improve and manage all aspects of an older persons' care, and may reduce adverse events in frail older adults, particularly when delivered in combination with complex interventions in community settings [15]. CGA is therefore a central component in the implementation of integrated care pathways (ICPs) to manage the care needs of older people. ICPs describe structured multidisciplinary care plans, detailing clear instructions for the management of patients [16]. It is suggested that these pathways may be useful in the treatment of frail older adults [17]. Although ICPs are increasingly being developed and validated in healthcare settings [18], few studies have confirmed their benefits in frailty [19].

In Ireland, few ICPs exist and to our knowledge none have been used in this setting. The Healy report [20], on community healthcare organisations in Ireland, called for the development of integrated healthcare, to strengthen the relationship between primary, secondary and social care. Another more recent report into integrated healthcare in Ireland has identified many challenges to implementing integrated care including policy and organisational barriers [21]. Combining ICPs with recent technological advances is postulated to facilitate the exchange of information and streamline clinical decision-makings [17], potentially overcoming these difficulties. Integrating information and communications technology (ICT) with screening and assessment is now recognised as a key facilitator to assist in the implementation of ICPs in clinical practice. Projects such as the FP-7 funded PERsonalised ICT Supported Service for Independent Living and Active Ageing (PERSSILAA, see www.perssilaa.eu), composed of partners from the EIP-AHA, identifies robust, pre-frail and frail older adults in the community, using ICT strategies to manage patients' cognitive, functional and nutritional domains [22]. However, there is a need to clearly define the type of interventions, the methods and outcomes applied [23] as well as which patients will benefit most. A systematic review of ICPs recommends that given budgetary constraints (cost of developing and implementing these), pathways should be restricted to areas with clearly identified deficiencies in existing care provision and/or where change is required [24]. Given this, there is a need to rationalise the delivery of ICPs in the community. Screening for those at the highest risk of adverse healthcare outcomes identifies those who may benefit most from interventions. A growing number of frailty assessment instruments, each with their own advantages and disadvantages are available [25], though no single instrument is recommended. More recently, it is suggested that as risk and frailty are closely related, specific risk-prediction instruments may be as useful in identifying and triaging frail older adults most likely to experience adverse healthcare outcomes [26–28].

2   The Community Assessment of Risk and Treatment Strategies (CARTS)

The Community Assessment of Risk and Treatment Strategies (CARTS), developed by the Centre for Gerontology and Rehabilitation (CGR) in University College Cork (UCC), Ireland, is a patient-centred ICP based upon an evidence-based screening and assessment programme (see http://www.ucc.ie/en/charge-ucc/carts/). The CARTS ICP model was included as one of three good practice initiatives in Irelands, successful reference site bid under the European Innovation Partnership on Active and Healthy Ageing (EIP-AHA), called the COLLoration on AGEing (COLLAGE), (see http://www.collage-ireland.eu/). COLLAGE [29, 30], formed from the merger of Irelands two initial reference site applications: The Cork Healthy Ageing through Resource Generation and Education programme (CHARGE), coordinated by UCC and the Louth Age Friendly County initiative, coordinated by NetwellCASALA, is involved in all six of the initial, specific, action groups projects under the EIP-AHA.

The CARTS programme was developed using the framework of the Medical Research Council for the development and evaluation of complex interventions [31].

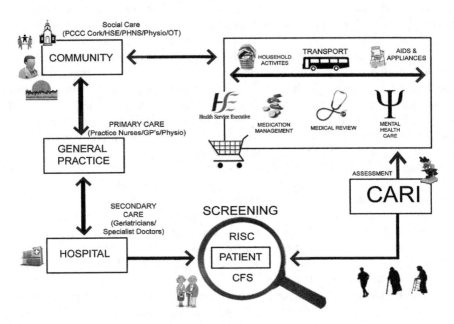

Fig. 1. Graphic representation of the Community Assessment of Risk and Treatment Strategies screening and assessment model.

(1) Development Phase: The concept of developing an ICP arose in 2011, when the CGR in UCC was approached by the local Primary, Community and Continuing Care (PCCC) team of the Health Service Executive of Ireland (HSE) to develop an instrument to evaluate the care needs of frail older people in the community. The existing tools available to community healthcare professionals (HCPs), such as community or public health nurses (PHNs), assessed characteristics of individuals but did not allow them to prioritise need or ensure appropriate allocation of services and resources. From this, CARTS developed into an intervention pathway to screen and triage patients according to risk of adverse healthcare outcomes, facilitated through the local PCCC in St Finbarr's Hospital, Cork. A literature review was conducted to establish best practice. A training package and manual for the CARTS programme was developed. To assess barriers to and facilitators of the implementation of an integrated screening and assessment programme in clinical practice, a questionnaire was sent to HCPs locally and focus groups were held with both hospital and community multi-disciplinary teams to discuss training packages, relevant predictors, suitable assessment instruments and interventions. Feedback was incorporated into the programme and a suite of new, short screening and assessment instruments were designed and

trialed specifically for use in the CARTS programme. These included a short, screening instrument, the Community Assessment of Risk Screening Instrument or CARST, now renamed the Risk Instrument for Screening in the Community (RISC) [27, 28, 32–36] and a short CGA instrument called the Community Assessment of Risk Instrument (CARI) [37]. Both were converted into computerised applications (apps) (Fig. 2).

(2) Feasibility phase: An initial audit of risk registers was conducted in public health centres in Cork, Ireland in 2011. Risk registers, designed to be used with HSE risk assessment tools, provide a composite of the likelihood and impact of adverse outcomes from one (remote and negligible) to five (almost certain with extreme impact), combined into a risk matrix. A subsequent audit established that approximately 7 % of these community-dwelling older adults were high-risk [38].

(3) Evaluation and Implementation: Since, considerable work has taken place in Ireland and other countries to develop the CARTS model, which now comprises of four stages (Fig. 3):

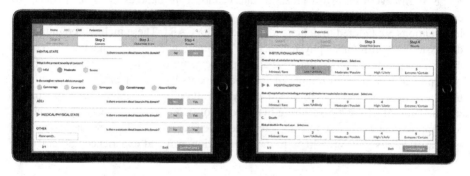

Fig. 2. Tablet computerised versions of the Community Assessment of Risk and Treatment Strategies (CARTS) instruments.

Stage 1: Screening. The RISC was developed and validated, as a brief screening instrument to measure risk of three adverse outcomes (institutionalisation, hospitalisation and death) in community dwelling older adults [27, 28]. The RISC is short (2–5 min), comprehensive, reliable [32], easy to administer and has high internal consistency [35]. It is used as a 'pre-screen', stratifying patients according to their risk level. It collects demographic data and identifies concern for three core domains: Mental State, ADL and Medical State. Each issue identified is graded in severity, from mild to severe, the effect of the care network is noted, and risk is determined such that: Risk equates to the severity of the concern minus the protective effect of the caregiver network. The RISC is available at http://www.biomedcentral.com/1471-2318/14/104/figure/F1. The RISC uniquely measures the ability of the caregiver network to manage risk [36]. It is scored as a five-point global subjective risk score from 1 to 5, where 1 is the lowest risk and 5 is the highest of an adverse healthcare outcome. Patients can be grouped into minimum (RISC scores 1 & 2), moderate (RISC score 3) and maximum-risk (RISC scores 4 & 5) to facilitate analysis. The RISC was initially validated in Ireland against the Clinical Frailty Scale (CFS) [4], a well-validated frailty instrument, in 803 community dwellers over 65 years. Those classified as maximum-risk were significantly more likely to experience outcomes at one year. The RISC had greater, albeit it was non-significant, accuracy than the CFS. Since, the RISC has been translated and piloted in several other countries (Spain, Portugal, Canada, Australia & the United Kingdom). The RISC validation was awarded the HSEs Lenus Open Access Research (Social Care) Award 2014.

Stage 2: Assessment. The CARI is a short (10 min), CGA proforma, completed on patients who screen positive on the RISC. The three core domains are further subdivided into sections and issues. Highlighted issues are then targeted with tailored interventions. The CARI, available at http://www.jfrailtyaging.com/all-issues.html? article=231, has good inter-rater reliability [37]. When inconsistencies occurred, they appeared to relate to differences in the professional background of the raters. These have led to the further development of the instrument. The CARI is also translated and validated in Ireland, Portugal and Spain.

Stage 3: Intervention. Most recently, intervention care bundles have been added to complement the delivery of the CARTS screening and assessment model. These interventions are tailored to deficits identified in the CARI. These include "cognition & depression", "nutrition", "physical activity", "function & falls", "medical", "continence", "sensory & pain", and "social support & environment" care bundles. These were piloted in a random sample of Irish participants (n = 10) identified as high-risk using the RISC screen (baseline and one year follow-up), compared with randomly matched controls (n = 30), resulting in a median of two referrals per participant, which took approximately 90 min to complete. After one year, the results were promising but not statistically significant: 30 % in the intervention arm had experienced at least one

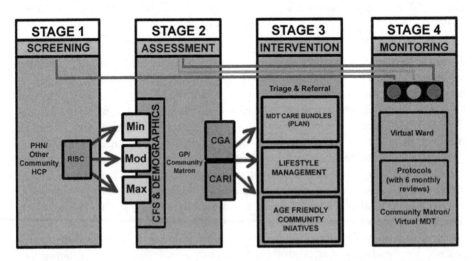

Fig. 3. The Community Assessment of Risk and Treatment Strategies (CARTS) integrated care pathway model.

Table 1. Studies demonstrating feasibility and utility of the Community Assessment of Risk and Treatment Strategies (CARTS) instruments and pilot.

Instrument	Study site	Year	Type	Sample	Outcome	Reference
Risk register	Ireland	2012	Audit of current practice	N=783	Prevalence of risk as captured by existing risk assessment	O'Caoimh N, Healy E, O'Connell E, Molloy D.W. Stratification of the Risk of Adverse Outcomes for Irish, Community Dwelling, Older Adults: Use of a Risk Register. *Irish Journal of Medical Science* 2012, 181 S(7) p295.
RISC (CARST)	Canada & Ireland	2012	Reliability	N=115	High inter-rater reliability and internal consistency	O'Caoimh N, Healy E, O'Connell E, Gao Y, Molloy D.W. The Community Assessment of Risk Tool. (CART); Investigation of Inter-Rater Reliability for a New Instrument measuring risk of Adverse Outcomes in Community Dwelling Older Adults. *Irish Journal of Medical Science* 2012,181 S(7) p227.
RISC & CPS	Ireland	2014	Validation	N=803	Accuracy compared to the CPS (frailty measure)	FitzGerald C, O'Caoimh R, Healy E, O'Keeffe G, Cronin U, O'Herlihy E, Cornally N, Clarnette R, Coveney S, Orfila F, Paul C, Lupari M, Molloy DW. Risk Instrument for Screening in the Community (RISC): Predicting Adverse Outcomes in Older Adults. *Irish Journal of Medical Science* 2014 183 S(7) p306-7. O'Caoimh R, Gao Y, Svendrovski A, Healy E, O'Connell E, O'Keeffe G, Cronin U, O'Herlihy E, Cornally N, Molloy DW. Screening for markers of frailty and perceived risk of adverse outcomes using the Risk Instrument for Screening in the Community (RISC). *BMC Geriatrics* 2014;14-104 doi:10.1186/1471-2318-14-104.
RISC	Ireland	2014	Validation	N=803	Survival analysis	O'Caoimh R, Gao Y, Svendrovski A, Healy E, O'Connell E, O'Keeffe G, Leahy-Warren P, Cronin U, O'Herlihy E, Cornally N, Molloy DW. The Risk Instrument for Screening in the Community (RISC); A New Instrument for Pre-dicting Risk of Adverse Outcomes in Community Dwelling Older Adults. *BMC Geriatrics*, 2015 Jul 30;15:92. doi: 10.1186/s12877-015-0095-z.
CARI	Australia	2014	Reliability & comparison to CGA	N=50	High inter-rater reliability and internal consistency	Clarnette RM, Ryan JF, O'Herlihy E, Svendrovski A, Cornally N, O'Caoimh R, Leahy-Warren P, Paul C, Molloy DW The Community Assessment of Risk Instrument: Investigation of Inter-Rater Reliability of an Instrument Measuring Risk of Adverse Outcomes: *Journal of Frailty and Aging* 2015 ;4(2):80-89
RISC	Ireland	2014	2° Analysis of the components, subtests and caregiver network scores	N=779	Accuracy of the caregiver network component was greater than other short measures e.g. Barthel Index	Leahy-Warren P, O'Caoimh R, Fitzgerald C, Cochrane A, Svendrovski A, Cronin U, O'Herlihy E, Cornally N, FitzGerald C, Gao Y, Healy E, O'Connell E, O'Keeffe G, Coveney S, McGlynn S, Clarnette R, Molloy DW Components of the Risk Instrument for Screening in the Community (RISC) that predict Public Health Nurse perception of risk. *Journal of Frailty & Aging* 2015;4(3):149-154. O'Caoimh R, FitzGerald C, Cronin U, Svendrovski A, Gao Y, Healy E, O'Connell E, O'Keeffe G, O'Herlihy E, Weathers E, Cornally N, Leahy-Warren P, Orfila F, Paul C, Clarnette R, Molloy DW. Which part of a short, global risk assessment, the Risk Instrument for Screening in the Community (RISC), predicts adverse healthcare outcomes? *Journal of Aging Research*, 2015 Article ID 256414, 7 pages. doi:10.1155/2015/256414. O'Caoimh R, FitzGerald C, Cronin U, Svendrovski A, Gao Y, Healy E, O'Connell E, O'Keeffe G, O'Herlihy E, Nicola Cornally N, Leahy-Warren P, Clarnette R, Molloy DW. The effect of caregiver networks in predicting patients' risk of adverse healthcare outcomes. *Irish Ageing Studies Review* 2015 6 (1) p318-319.
RISC	Spain, Portugal, Northern Ireland, Australia & Ireland	2014	Qualitative analysis	N=28	Cross cultural perspectives	Leahy-Warren P, Weathers E, Lupari M, Campbell S, Clarnette R, Orfila F, Fitzgerald C, Paul C, O'Herlihy E, Cornally N, O'Caoimh R, Day MR, Mulcahy H, Kropmans TJ. Risk Instrument for Screening Older People in the Community (RISC): Cross Cultural Perspectives. Submitted to the *International Journal of Research in Nursing* 2015. DOI: 10.3844/ijrnsp.2015
RISC	Portugal	2014	Prevalence study	N=2,125	Baseline demographics, risk profile in Portugal	Paul C, Teixeira L, Azevedo MJ, Alves S, Duarte M, O'Caoimh R, Molloy W. Risk of mental health problems in primary care. Submitted Frontiers in Neuroscience under re-review 2015.
RISC	Spain	2014	Prevalence study & on-going validation	N=574	Baseline demographics, risk profile in Spain	Orfila F, Cegri F, Canela M, Heserqui P, Cox S, Peligros X, Molloy DW. Proyecto CARTS; estudio piloto de una herramienta de riesgo de fragilidad y declive funcional en la personas mayores en Atención Primaria. 4a Jornada del Pla de Salut de Cataluyna 2011-2015. Sitges, 28 noviembre 2014.
CARTS Interventions	Ireland	2014-2015	Pilot case control study	N=40	Risk reduction in adverse se outcomes at one year	Outcomes for the Community Assessment of Risk & Treatment Strategies study. Accepted for *Gerontological Society of America* conference November 2015
CARTS risk screens	NA	NA	Systematic review	NA	Overview of risk prediction instruments	O'Caoimh R, Cornally N, Weathers E, O'Sullivan R, Fitzgerald C, Orfila F, Clarnette R, Paul C, Molloy DW. Risk prediction in the community: A systematic review of case-finding instruments that predict adverse healthcare outcomes in community dwelling older adults. *Maturitas* September 2015, 82; (1)-3-21
CARTS ICP	EIP-AHA reference site of COLLAGE-role of CARTS	NA	NA	Integrated review	NA	Overview of CARTS ICP	Sweeney C, Molloy DW, O'Caoimh R, Bond R, Hynes H, McGuade C, Cornally N, Daly E et al. COLLaboration on AGEing-COLLAGE: Ireland's three star reference site for the European Innovation Partnership on Active and Healthy Ageing: *Irish Journal of Medical Science* 2013, 182 S(6) p278-279. O'Caoimh R, Sweeney C, Hynes H, McGuade C, Cornally N, Daly E et al. COLLaboration on AGEing-COLLAGE: Ireland's three star reference site for the European Innovation Partnership on Active and Healthy Ageing (EIP on AHA). *European Geriatric Medicine* 2015 DOI: 10.1159/000413432. Weathers EJ, O'Caoimh R, Paul C, Clarnette R, Orfila F, O'Sullivan R, Daly BO, Cornally N, Molloy DW. The Community Assessment of Risk Screening and Treatment Strategies (CARTS) programme: An Update. *ICT4Ageing Well* 2015 Lisbon, Portugal 20-22 May 2015.

adverse outcome compared to 35.5 % of controls (Fisher's Exact test one-tailed p-value = 0.535).

Stage 4. Monitoring. The final stage of the CARTS model is interval monitoring. The computerised app is used to facilitate monitoring using a traffic light system (See Figs. 1 and 3). Publications, conference abstracts and peer-reviewed full papers are presented in Table 1.

3 Impact of the CARTS Programme

The CARTS programme has the potential to significantly impact on (1) older people, (2) healthcare providers and (3) healthcare services (Fig. 3).

3.1 Older Adults

For an older adult living in the community, the expected outcomes of CARTS are:

- A reduced incidence of frailty in pre-frail or robust older adults, potentially showing reversal in those already frail and transition states e.g. from pre-frail to robust.
- An extended length of time in relative functional independence in their preferred home or care setting (reduced incidence in institutionalisation).
- The maintenance of a safe level of ADL and ambulation leading to a reduction in falls and hence injuries.
- Reduced susceptibility to acute illness, which may lead to adverse outcomes (e.g. falls, institutionalisation, hospitalisation and death).
- Knowledge of likely outcomes and then appropriate planning (patients in all groups will be provided with lifestyle advice).
- Better management and reduction of multiple comorbidities.
- Empower patients and caregivers by warning them of their risk profile and possible interventions to minimise risk (patients and carers will be informed of their RISC score and frailty status).
- Increased satisfaction and quality of life (QOL); key outcome measures of the success of ICPs.

3.2 Healthcare Providers

For healthcare providers (GPs, PHNs, HSE General Managers, Consultant Geriatricians, Nurse Educators etc.), the potential impact includes:

- Improved assessment, identification and management of older frail adults.
- Enhanced documentation and communication of the older person's functional capacity, interventions used and outcomes.
- Provision of integrated care across a network of community nurses, primary care practitioners, and specialists in secondary and tertiary care.

3.3 Healthcare Systems

For healthcare services and wider society, CARTS has the potential to:

- Show the potential that simple ICT systems have in providing integrated care, reducing organisational barriers.
- Increase more appropriate targeted assessment across settings; facilitating greater integration between community services, family doctors, and hospitals with a strong primary care focus at its centre, which is known to produce better health outcomes at lower costs.
- Enable prompt and accurate referral for evaluation of frailty, potentially reducing waiting lists, length of stay and delayed discharge; potentially reducing demand on nursing homes and hospitals by this high-risk group.
- Increase early utilisation of rehabilitative services (e.g. cognitive rehabilitation, occupational and physical therapy).
- Support institutional policies/programmes that promote function e.g. caregiver educational efforts and walking programmes etc.
- Provide evidence of continued interdisciplinary assessments and care evaluation.

4 External Validation of the CARTS ICP

Recently, work to translate and externally validate the CARTS programme has been undertaken in several countries including Portugal, Spain, Australia, and most recently the United Kingdom (Northern Ireland). The RISC and CARI were validated in Spain, Portugal and Australia. Validation of the instruments in Australia and Spain is complete and being prepared for publication. In Portugal, baseline data collection is complete and has been submitted for publication although outcome data is still awaited. Contrasts between these different healthcare systems present challenges when piloting the CARTS ICP model.

4.1 Portugal

In Portugal, Family Health Units (FHU), self-selecting groups, made up of 3–8 GPs, family nurses and administrative staff, deliver primary care to approximately half of registered patients. FHUs consistently outperform the pre-existing Primary Health Care Units, showing the potential of ICPs in Portugal. In 2007, the National Network of Integrated Continuous Care was established to integrate health and social services for older adults requiring long term care in Portugal and in 2013, plans for the development of ICPs were introduced. However, their implementation faces financial and political challenges, limiting their utility [39]. Since its introduction into the Porto Metropolitan area, the CARTS ICP model has been used to screen community-dwelling older adults for risk of adverse outcomes. In Portugal, 4499 community-dwelling older adults have been screened using the RISC and are currently being followed [40]. The sample consisted of 1854 (41.2 %) males and 2645 (58.8 %) females with a mean age of 76.3 years (standard deviation = +/–7.3, range = 65–103 years). Only 734 patients (16.7 %)

were living alone. In total, 1616 (35.9 %) of the patients were scored as having mental health concerns using the RISC, compared with 2043 (45.4 %) with ADL concerns and 3222 (78.3 %) with medical concerns. Of patients with mental health concerns on the RISC, less than half (48.5 %) had a caregiver network that was perceived to be able to manage the situation. Evaluating the risk of adverse outcomes showed that 16.3 % of the sample was perceived to be at risk of institutionalisation, 32.8 % at risk of hospitalisation and 23.1 % at risk of death [40].

4.2   Spain

In Spain, different models of integration are emerging. Two main approaches can be distinguished: one that focuses on clinical processes (micro level), and another on the organizational architecture of the health delivery system (meso-macro level). Work in Spain is presently focused on integrated care for patients with multiple chronic conditions or complex disease management [41]. In Catalonia, the *Chronicity Prevention and Care Programme*, substituting traditional face-to-face care with transfer and shared responsibilities between patients, citizens and health care professionals has reduced the rate of emergency admissions and readmission related to chronic conditions and improved outcomes relating to better chronic disease control [42]. In Barcelona, 374 community-dwelling older adults included in Home Care were screened using the RISC and followed for one year to confirm the predictive validity of the translated version. A translated computerised application is also being used (see Fig. 4). Results showed that 48.4 % had mental problems, 93.6 % had problems with activities of daily living, and 80 % medical/physical problems [43]. With regards to the caregiver network, 20.6 % of caregivers were burdened and 24.1 % had problems or couldn't handle the situation. Overall, there were 19.3 % who had a high risk of developing adverse outcomes in the next year, with 8.6 % at high risk of institutionalisation, 13.4 % at high risk of hospitalisation and 7.2 % at high risk of death [43]. There were statistically significant associations between being at high risk of adverse outcomes and other morbidity measures such as worse Clinical Risk Groups classification, being a complex or advanced chronic patient, having chronic obstructive pulmonary disease, dementia and a high score on the Barthel Index. Problems with the ability of the caregiver network to cope were also associated with higher risk of adverse outcomes [43]. Those in the maximum risk category were almost 3 times more likely to be institutionalised at one year compared to those in the minimum risk group (16 % versus 6 %, p = 0.002). These trends were also found for one-year risk of death (33.3 % versus 13.2 % P < 0.001) but not hospitalisation (24.2 % versus 17.3 %, p = 0.10). The RISC had fair accuracy for risk of death (area under the curve of 0.70) and institutionalisation (area under the curve of 0.66) but again had weak accuracy for hospitalisation (area under the curve of 0.55).

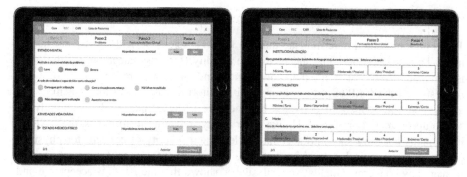

Fig. 4. Spanish translated version of the CARTS instruments.

4.3 Australia

In Australia, over 500 community-dwelling older adults have been screened using the RISC and the CARI completed as part of a formalised CGA. Inter-rater reliability in a sample of 50 patients was assessed by a nurse and a doctor [37]. The instrument was found to have good reliability across all domains, especially for risk of death and institutionalisation. Following receipt of a grant from the Fremantle Hospital Medical Research Foundation, the Australian cohort is now undergoing 12-month analysis for the three key outcomes of hospitalisation, institutionalisation and death.

5 Challenges and Solutions for Scaling-up CARTS

Given that CARTS is being piloted in disparate study sites and in different languages, socio-technical issues relating to differences in cultural practice and organisational factors between the countries are foreseen and need to be accounted for. This section details work already completed in an attempt to account for the social, cultural and political context of the project. Preliminary work comparing the baseline demographics and RISC data between countries participating in the CARTS project highlights the challenges with undertaking up-scaling of projects in different countries. The experiences of HCPs who have used the screening pathway with community-dwelling older adults in the three study countries included in this project were surveyed in focus groups [44]. As different HCPs can perform screening, persons from a variety of disciplines were sampled including Geriatricians, General Practitioners (GPs), PHNs, registered practice nurses and social workers. Several operational challenges were identified and recommendations for improvement made. Cultural differences were found between participants with regards to terminologies such as 'caregiver network' and 'insight' and expectation in relation to caring. Interdisciplinary differences were also identified related to different conceptualisations of health. Based upon these, cultural, institutional and language adjustments were made to the translated versions of the RISC and CARI.

6 Conclusion

The results presented here indicate that the CARTS screening and assessment instruments have good concurrent and predictive validity (for hospitalisation, institutionalisation and death), high internal consistency and inter-rater reliability. Pilot work suggests that the CARTS interventions and monitoring will add to the screening and assessment components to deliver a holistic care pathway that could potentially be scaled up in Ireland or abroad. Unlike other frailty screening instruments, the CARTS instruments not only take into account the level and severity of concern for physical, cognitive and medical conditions but also the ability of the caregiver network to manage any concerns. Qualitative analysis has shown that the RISC is acceptable and applicable cross-culturally [44] and pilot studies of translated versions (Spanish and Portuguese) suggest that the approach can be used to screen and triage in different countries and cultures with minimal effort. This cross-border applicability suggests that the CARTS ICP may be scaled up, making it of relevance to EU policy-makers. Research is now needed to validate the CARTS instruments in other languages and show the utility of incorporating the CARTS intervention care bundles into the screening and assessment components to make a truly valid beneficial ICP to manage frailty and frailty transitions in community-dwelling older adults.

7 Future Development of the CARTS Project

As part of the EIP-AHA star ceremony in 2013, the CARTS programme was awarded three stars (highest rating) contributing to the designation of the Irish reference site, COLLAGE, as a three star reference site for active and healthy ageing. The research team in Ireland plan to apply for funding to scale up the CARTS ICP model in different EU sites. The CARTS data will continue to be collected as a component of comprehensive geriatric assessment in Western Australia to the two-year time point. Analysis of the first 12 months of risk outcomes is nearly complete and will continue at the 12-month and 24 month time points. The next phase of the project will focus on the initial RISC rating followed by comparison to rating at the time of subsequent CGA. In Spain, funding has been obtained from the Primary Care Office of the Catalan Health Institute to conduct a follow-up of the pilot study and to train 15 more nurses and screen 500 more community-dwelling older adults. In March 2015, an application was submitted for national funding (Carlos III Institute, Madrid) in collaboration with the Irish team, to validate the CARTS programme and conduct a RCT study. The first phase of this study will screen and follow a cohort of 2000 people with the RISC and the second phase will compare a medium-high risk group, receiving the CARTS intervention, to a matched control group, receiving the usual standard of care. In Portugal, the Directorate-General of Health, Portuguese Ministry of Health together with the University of Porto financed CARTS as part of the screening phase of Primary Care patients with mental health disorders.

In summary, the CARTS programme seeks to keep older adults healthy, independent and active in their own homes and to link and integrate social and medicine services between the patient and caregiver network in the community, with family doctors and specialty clinics. In doing so, it is expected that the programme will provide both clinical and economic benefits. The impact of the programme will be clearly measured from these aspects. The programme will be of mutual benefit to the individual and society from a health and economic perspective. Person-centred, care protocols will be targeted to older adults in accordance with their needs in primary healthcare systems. For older persons living in the community, CARTS aims to reduce the risk of adverse outcomes including institutionalisation and death through early intervention, and improve patient quality of life. This research is important for healthcare providers as it provides a framework to identify high-risk older adults and intervene early. This research is also important for health policymakers, as it uses a preventive approach to community healthcare and strengthens service integration. The strength of the CARTS programme is in its scalability and ability to evaluate evidence-based care pathways for individuals in a quick, easy manner. The use of ICT should facilitate this scaling up and help drive forward the delivery of ICPs such as the CARTS programme in clinical practice.

References

1. Rachel, B., et al.: Ageing in the European union. Lancet **381**(9874), 1312–1322 (2013)
2. Clegg, A., et al.: Frailty in elderly people. Lancet **381**(9868), 752–762 (2013). Accessed 2 March 2013
3. Prince, M.J., Wu, F., Guo, Y.F., Robledo, L.M.G., O'Donnell, M., Sullivan, R., Yusuf, S.: The burden of disease in older people and implications for health policy and practice. Lancet **385**, 549–562 (2015)
4. Rockwood, K., et al.: A global clinical measure of fitness and frailty in elderly people. CMAJ **173**(5), 489–495 (2005). Accessed 30 August 2005
5. Collard, R.M., Boter, H., Schoevers, R.A., Oude Voshaar, R.C.: Prevalence of frailty in community-dwelling older persons: a systematic review. J AM Geriatr. Soc. **60**(8), 1487–1492 (2012)
6. Van Rensbergen, G., Nawrot, T.: Medical conditions of nursing home admissions. BMC Geriatr. **10**(1), 46 (2010)
7. Khandelwal, D., Goel, A., Kumar, U., Gulati, V., Narang, R., Dey, A.B.: Frailty is associated with longer hospital stay and increased mortality in hospitalized older patients. J. Nutr. Health Aging **16**(8), 732–735 (2012)
8. Chang, S.F., Lin, P.L.: Frail phenotype and mortality prediction: a systematic review and meta-analysis of prospective cohort studies. Int. J. Nurs. Stud. (2015, in press)
9. Kulmala, J., Nykänen, I., Hartikainen, S.: Frailty as a predictor of all-cause mortality in older men and women. Geriatr. Gerontol. Int. **14**(4), 899–905 (2014)
10. Chang, Y.-W., et al.: Frailty and its impact on health-related quality of life: a cross-sectional study on elder community-dwelling preventive health service users. PLoS ONE **7**(5), e38079 (2012). doi:10.1371/journal.pone.0038079
11. Fassbender, K., Fainsinger, R.L., Carson, M., Finegan, B.A.: Cost trajectories at the end of life: the Canadian experience. J. Pain Symptom Manag. **38**(1), 75–80 (2009)
12. Robinson, T.N., et al.: Frailty predicts increased hospital and six-month healthcare cost following colorectal surgery in older adults. Am. J. Surg. **202**(5), 511–514 (2011)

13. Rodríguez-Mañas, L., Féart, C., Mann, G., et al.: Searching for an operational definition of frailty: a delphi method based consensus statement: the frailty operative definition-consensus conference project. J. Gerontol. A Biol. Sci. Med. Sci. **68**, 62–67 (2013)

14. Gordon, A.L., et al.: Now that we have a definition for physical frailty, what shape should frailty medicine take? Age Ageing **2014**(43), 8–9 (2014)

15. Beswick, A.D., et al.: Complex interventions to improve physical function and maintain independent living in elderly people: a systematic review and meta-analysis. Lancet **371**, 725–735 (2008)

16. Campbell, H., Hotchkiss, R., Bradshaw, N., Porteous, M.: Integrated care pathways. BMJ **316**, 133 (1998)

17. Dubuc, N., Bonin, L., Tourigny, A., Mathieu, L., Couturier, Y., Tousignant, M., Corbin, C., Delli-Colli, N., Raîche, M.: Development of integrated care pathways: toward a care management system to meet the needs of frail and disabled community-dwelling older people. Int. J. Integr. Care **13**, e017 (2013)

18. Sun, X., Tang, W., Ye, T., Zhang, Y., Wen, B., Zhang, L.: Integrated care: a comprehensive bibliometric analysis and literature review. Int. J. Integr. Care. **14**, e017. eCollection (2014). Accessed 12 June 2014

19. Bendayan, M., et al.: Therapeutic interventions for frail elderly patients: part II. Ongoing and unpublished randomized trials. Prog. Cardiovasc. Dis. **57**(2), 144–51 (2014)

20. Healy, P.: Community healthcare organisations - report and recommendations of the integrated service area review group [internet]. Health Service Executive, Dublin, October 2014. http://www.hse.ie/eng/services/publications/corporate/CHOReport.html

21. Darker, C.: Integrated healthcare in Ireland – a critical analysis and a way forward: an adelaide health foundation policy paper (2014). http://www.adelaide.ie/Wp-content/uploads/2015/01/integrated-Healthcare-in-ireland.pdf. Accessed 16 September 2015

22. van Velsen, L., Illario, M., et al.: A community-based, technology-supported health service for detecting and preventing frailty among older adults: a participatory design development process. J. Aging Res. **2015**, Article ID 216084, 9 (2015). doi:10.1155/2015/216084

23. Vanhaecht, K., Ovretveit, J., Elliott, M.J., Sermeus, W., Ellershaw, J., Panella, M.: Have we drawn the wrong conclusions about the value of care pathways? Is a Cochrane review appropriate? Eval. Health Prof. **35**(1), 28–42 (2012)

24. Allen, D., Gillen, E., Rixson, L.: Systematic review of the effectiveness of integrated care pathways: what works, for whom, in which circumstances? Int. J. Evid. Based Healthc. **7**(2), 61–74 (2009)

25. de Vries, N.M., Staal, J.B., van Ravensberg, C.D., Hobbelen, J.S.M., Olde Rikkerte, M.G.M., Nijhuis-van der Sanden, M.W.G.: Outcome instruments to measure frailty: a systematic review. Ageing Res. Rev. **10**, 104–114 (2011)

26. O'Caoimh, R., Cornally, N., Weathers, E., O'Sullivan, R., Fitzgerald, C., Orfila, F., Clarnette, R., Paúl, C., Molloy, D.W.: Risk prediction in the community: a systematic review of case-finding instruments that predict adverse healthcare outcomes in community-dwelling older adults. Maturitas **82**(1), 3–21 (2015)

27. O'Caoimh, R., Gao, Y., Svendrovski, A., Healy, E., O'Connell, E., O'Keeffe, G., Cronin, U., O'Herlihy, E., Cornally, N., Molloy, D.W.: Screening for markers of frailty and perceived risk of adverse outcomes using the risk instrument for screening in the community (RISC). BMC Geriatr. **14**, 104 (2014). doi:10.1186/1471-2318-14-104

28. O'Caoimh, R., Gao, Y., Svendrovski, A., Healy, E., O'Connell, E., O'Keeffe, G., Leahy-Warren, P., Cronin, U., O'Herlihy, E., Cornally, N., Molloy, D.W.: The risk instrument for screening in the community (RISC): a new instrument for predicting risk of adverse outcomes in community dwelling older adults. BMC Geriatr. **15**, 92 (2015). doi:10.1186/s12877-015-0095-z. Accessed 30 July 2015

29. Sweeney, C., Molloy, D.W., O'Caoimh, R., Bond, R., Hynes, H., McGlade, C., Shorten, G.: European innovation partnership on active and healthy ageing: Ireland and the COLLAGE experience. Irish J. Med. Sci. **182**(S(6)), 278–279 (2015)

30. O'Caoimh, R., Sweeney, C., Hynes, H., McGlade, C., Cornally, N., Daly, E., et al.: COLLaboration on AGEing-COLLAGE: Ireland's three star reference site for the European innovation partnership on active and healthy ageing (EIP on AHA). Eur. Geriatr. Med. (2015). doi:10.1159/000433432

31. Craig, P., et al.: Developing and evaluating complex interventions: the new medical research council guidance. BMJ **337**(7676), 979–983 (2008)

32. O'Caoimh, R., Healy, E., O' Connell, E., Gao, Y., Molloy, D.W.: The community assessment of risk tool (CART): investigation of inter-rater reliability for a new instrument measuring risk of adverse outcomes in community dwelling older adults. Irish J. Med. Sci. **181**(S(7)), 227 (2012)

33. FitzGerald, C., O'Caoimh, R., Healy, E., O'Connell, E., O'Keeffe, G., Cronin, U., O'Herlihy, E., Cornally, N., Clarnette, R., Coveney, S., Orfila, F., Paul, C., Lupari, M., Molloy, D.W.: Risk instrument for screening in the community (RISC): predicting adverse outcomes in older adults. Irish J. Med. Sci. **183**(S7), 306–307 (2014)

34. Leahy-Warren, P., O'Caoimh, R., Fitzgerald, C., Cochrane, A., Svendrovski, A., Cronin, U., O'Herlihy, E., Cornally, N., FitzGerald, C., Gao, Y., Healy, E., O'Connell, E., O'Keeffe, G., Coveney, S., McGlynn, J., Clarnette, R., Molloy, D.W.: Components of the risk instrument for screening in the community (RISC) that predict public health nurse perception of risk. J. Frailty Aging **4**(3), 149–154 (2015)

35. O'Caoimh, R., FitzGerald, C., Cronin, U., Svendrovski, A., Gao, Y., Healy, E., O'Connell, E., O'Keeffe, G., O'Herlihy, E., Weathers, E., Cornally, N., Leahy-Warren, P., Orfila, F., Paúl, C., Clarnette, R., Molloy, D.W.: Which part of a short, global risk assessment, the risk instrument for screening in the community (RISC), predicts adverse healthcare outcomes? J. Aging Res. Article ID 256414, 7 (2015). doi:10.1155/2015/256414

36. O'Caoimh, R., FitzGerald, C., Cronin, U., Svendrovski, A., Gao, Y., Healy, E., O'Connell, E., O'Keeffe, G., O'Herlihy, E., Nicola Cornally, N., Leahy-Warren, P., Clarnette, R., Molloy, D.W.: The effect of caregiver networks in predicting patients' risk of adverse healthcare outcomes. Irish Ageing Stud. Rev. **6**(1), 318–319 (2015)

37. Clarnette, R.M., Ryan, J.P., O' Herlihy, E., Svendrovski, A., Cornally, N., O'Caoimh, R., Leahy-Warren, P., Paul, C., Molloy, D.W.: The community assessment of risk instrument: investigation of inter-rater reliability of an instrument measuring risk of adverse outcomes. J. Frailty Aging **4**(2), 80–89 (2015)

38. O'Caoimh, R., Healy, E., O' Connell, E., Molloy, D.W.: Stratification of the risk of adverse outcomes for Irish, community dwelling, older adults: use of a risk register. Irish J. Med. Sci. **181**(S7), 295 (2012)

39. Santana, S., et al.: Integration of care systems in Portugal: anatomy of recent reforms. Int. J. Integr. Care **14**, e014 (2014). PMID: 25114663

40. Paúl, C., Teixeira, L., Azevedo, M.J., Alves, S., Duarte, M., O'Caoimh, R, Molloy, W.: Perceived risk of mental health problems in primary care. Aging Neurosci. **7**, 212 (2015). doi:10.3389/fnagi.2015.00212

41. Nuño, R., et al.: Integrated care initiatives in the Spanish Health System: Abstracts from the Third Spanish Conference on Chronic Care, San Sebastián, 19–20 May 2011. Int. J. Integr. Care **12**(Suppl 2), e35 (2012). Accessed 29 May 2012

42. Contel, J.C., et al.: Chronic and integrated care in Catalonia. Int. J. Integr. Care **15**, e025 (2015)

43. Orfila, F., Cegri, F., Canela, M., Ensenyat, P., Cos, X., Peligros, X., Molloy, D.W.: Proyecto CARTS, estudio piloto de una herramienta de riesgo de fragilidad y declive funcional en la personas mayores en Atención Primaria. 4a Jornada del Pla de Salut de Catalunya 2011–2015. Sitges (2014). Accessed 28 noviembre 2014

44. Leahy-Warren, P., Weathers, E., Lupari, M., Campbell, S., Clarnette, R., Orfila, F., Fitzgerald, C., Paúl, C., O'Herlihy, E., Cornally, N., O'Caoimh, R., Day, M.R., Mulcahy, H., Molloy, D.W.: Risk instrument for screening older people in the community (RISC): cross cultural perspectives. Submitted Int. J. Res. Nurs. (2015). doi:10.3844/ijrnsp.2015

Advancing Ambient Assisted Living with Caution

Christian Huyck[1]([✉]), Juan Augusto[2], Xiaohong Gao[1], and Juan A. Botía[3]

[1] Artificial Intelligence Research Group, London, UK
c.huyck@mdx.ac.uk
[2] Research Group on Development of Intelligent Environments,
Middlesex University, London, UK
[3] Medical and Molecular Genetics, King's College London, London, UK
juan.botia@kcl.ac.uk

Abstract. As technology advances, systems involving artificial components provide more and more support for people. The potential consequences of this phenomena are examined in the specific circumstances of 'ambient assisted living' as an instantiation of the concept of 'intelligent environment'. This chapter describes the idea of 'ambient assisted living' and looks at some of the possible ways humans may be affected by the prevalence of technology. The general example of assisted healthcare, and the specific example of medication support are used to show that systems are advancing. Moreover, these advancements can lead to problems with both the artificial systems, and the larger systems with which they are involved. In many cases there is a trade-off around having people in the loop, but inevitably they will need to be included for many decision making processes. Keeping a person in the loop might also partially redress problems of Artificial General Intelligence systems. The chapter concludes with reflections on how these considerations can help us to retain the positive aspects whilst avoiding the negative side effects of the hypothetical technological singularity.

Keywords: Ambient Intelligence · Ambient assisted living · Human in the loop

1 Introduction

Artificial systems will become more sophisticated and will assist humans in more ways. While technology becomes more prevalent, it is important to guard against damages that this technology can cause [1]. Instead of blindly using more and more technology, it is important to consider problems that may arise from new technology

Artificial Intelligence is one set of technologies that is being used to support people. It is ill-defined, but generally refers to computer based systems that have a certain degree of intelligence. The systems can be used to help people in a wide range of tasks including robotics, Internet search, and language translation.

© Springer International Publishing Switzerland 2015
M. Helfert et al. (Eds.): ICT4AgeingWell 2015, CCIS 578, pp. 19–32, 2015.
DOI: 10.1007/978-3-319-27695-3_2

The state of the art in Artificial Intelligence is that domain specific systems can be built, but the systems are brittle and do not extend beyond the specific domain for which they were designed [2,3]. That does not mean the systems cannot learn, indeed learning is perhaps the major recent advancement in the area. Instead the systems fail altogether when they go beyond their intended purpose.

Ambient Intelligence foresees information systems in a way in which the user is the central entity [4]. By "Ambient Intelligence" we understand the intelligence embedded in an environment that is capable of understanding when humans can be assisted, deciding what type of assistance to offer and in which way to offer it, and if the users of that environment accepts this proposed assistance, then the system also has to deliver that assistance in the best possible way. By environments here we refer mainly to a physical space, typically a room or a building, although these systems can be deployed in less structured places. Examples of environments include a smart home, a smart office, a smart shopping mall, a plane, and a car. A surveillance system can operate in a street of the city, and a motorway can be equipped with sensing equipment to improve traffic conditions. In a smart home the system can collect information on the inhabitants, understand their whereabouts and routines and offer reminders and guidance with some tasks. In a smart office system, employees can be assisted by the system in managing information and documents so that they are better informed with less effort. A smart shopping mall can collect customer's preferences, advise customers on potentially interesting offers and shop owners on customers' reactions to certain items. Planes and cars are nowadays packed with sensing and actuating equipment that frequently takes decisions on behalf of the pilot or driver. These decisions are related to a diversity of areas, from fuel efficiency to safety in certain weather conditions. A street surveillance system can provide automatic detection of anti-social behaviour. Europe is already investing in improving road infrastructure so that the road can inform drivers about road conditions ahead; this interaction can also be between cars sharing data and increasing awareness of each others intentions and a municipality can use road use statistics to redirect users and optimize traffic.

In consequence, the technology is oriented towards (1) natural implicit interaction between the system and humans, (2) ubiquitous and smaller hardware disguised within the environment and (3) intelligent and autonomous behaviour. All the examples provided above have in common that the system in question provides assistance about daily life matters in exchange for being able to "observe" our daily life and gather a substantial amount of data. It seems that the more data the system can gather the more help the system should be able to offer. If a system has a record of what issues are important for the users and also of the subtle preferences the user has then it can not only realize that the user has not yet taken certain medicine and it will be useful to issue a reminder of that, but also to distinguish that as the user is talking to someone it needs to wait for a while. Clearly the other side of this coin is how this detailed knowledge of the user relates to privacy. There are other dimensions which are also very relevant to this chapter, for example, the dynamics created between the system and the users. Some users have different levels or receptiveness or rejection of systems which try to guide them. For those who are more accepting there are benefits, but sometimes dangers. By following the navigation system literally, you may drive against the traffic flow. This is especially feasible as these systems may reach a point where they provide reasonable advice for substantial periods of time, which leads to an assumption of perfection. We humans are usually keen on some sort of inertial thinking which suggests that things will go as usual unless something strange makes us think otherwise. When we turn the car on in the morning we assume it will work. Similarly in all these different environments, if the ambient system has been providing sensible advice about clever purchases, when to take medicines, which road to follow, which actions our company should be investing on, etc. we may get used to accept such advice as reasonable and gradually 'numbing' our critical processing of that interaction with the system.

This general concept becomes more specific when directed through application domains. One of the application domains of Ambient Intelligence is Ambient Assisted Living (AAL)[1]. AAL pursues the development of Information and Communication Technology (ICT) systems supporting independent daily living for people that may have a limited capacity to take care of themselves autonomously. Those AAL systems (AALSs), with an assistive orientation, are designed to ease daily tasks such as cooking, cleaning the house, having medication and social relationships. Moreover, such assistive focus is not only directed by the attended subject but also to family, caregivers and any other stakeholders within the global information system in which the AALS is subsumed (e.g. a care organization's health information system (HIS)). An example of an assistive task for the family is making them aware of up to date information about the subject's health condition through continuously monitoring the subject at home. Similarly, with respect to caregivers, they benefit from an AALS thanks to ubiquitous access to the subject's state at any time and anywhere. This considerably improves efficiency in their daily working routines. Thus an AALS works for different user roles and all these roles get some benefit in this relation.

The development of more and more intelligent and autonomous AALSs will, arguably, raise problems of a different nature. If they can be foreseen, solutions to these problems may be found.

While the authors of this chapter feel that it is unlikely that an Artificial General Intelligence (AGI) will be created by 2045 [5,6], we feel that considerations to prevent problems from AGIs would be both consistent with advances in AALSs and would benefit AALSs. For instance, checks and balances [7] should be used on AALSs to assure that they are supporting people appropriately. The authors also support both top-down and bottom-up controls of AALSs [8] to assure safe behaviour. Finally, keeping people in the loop not only reduces possible problems from AGIs, but is crucial for AALSs because people have the final authority in many decisions.

---

[1] http://www.aal-europe.eu/.

This chapter will focus on one particular AALS task: taking medicine. The scenario will be discussed in Sect. 2, and systems that currently support medicine taking will be addressed in Sect. 3. The chapter then engages in analysing, in a speculative manner, the different paths that advances in this technology might follow in the near future, exploring how the technology might advance, Sect. 4, and the more distant future, Sect. 5; these sections explore the technology, possible problems, and possible solutions to these problems. A brief Sect. 6 concludes.

2   Scenario

AAL is a vast field ranging from automatic setting of household temperature levels to cutting edge smart-rooms [9] that support education (see Sect. 3.1). A particularly active area within AAL is assisted healthcare (see Sect. 3.2.) The scenario explored below, from the area of assisted healthcare, is for technology to support people in taking medication. Taking medication is often important for people and in many cases crucial for them to live a normal life (see Sect. 3.2).

There are also a range of factors involved in taking medication. These include, but are by no means limited to, frequency of dose, regularity of that dose, dosage, combination with other medications, and if the medication is taken with or without food. Furthermore, a patient's adherence to the prescribed therapy is important as a high percentage of the people under treatment does not stick to the prescribed therapy. An important part of the group simply do not care about taking the medication, others may not even fill the prescription.

People have, of course, been taking medication from time immemorial. While they typically take the medication correctly, every person can make mistakes. People with learning disabilities, or short-term memory impairments can have particular difficulties. Technology already supports medication taking; for example, an alarm on a person's phone or watch can remind them to take their pill. Furthermore, other social factors, including cost of medication, can lead to a failure to take medication. There is scope to improve this further with systems actually monitoring whether tablets are taken, and potentially determining whether medication is needed at all.

3   State of the Art in Ambient Assisted Living

Currently, the AAL field is experiencing important advances, both in academia and industry, towards commercially available and dependable AALS products. There are particular applications in the health domain, and specific applications to support medicine taking. These systems are not perfect, but there are potentially solutions for some of their current problems.

3.1   Ambient Assisted Living

Nowadays, the main AAL target group of users is elderly people [10]. This is a natural consequence of the number of elderly people that keeps growing year by year worldwide. To cope with this scenario, governments focus an important part of their research programs on this broad community of users. A clear example of this is the AAL JP[2], an initiative of the European Commission devoted to funding research projects on using ICT to develop elder oriented AALSs[3]. For the same reason, companies see an interesting business possibility when focused on the elderly. However, AAL is oriented also to user groups with other kinds of impairments (e.g. mobility, visual, mental, and social).

An AAL ICT system is composed of a set of hardware and software elements. Hardware does not refer exclusively to personal computers, laptops, smartphones or tablets. It also includes any kind of sensor and actuator. Examples of sensors include room temperature, humidity, flood, and gas sensors; and wearable sensors such as body temperature, blood pressure or any sensor that might be relevant to perceiving part of the user context. Actuators are any device or appliance intended to modify the user's state. Examples of actuators range from simple automatic light switches to all the engines required to put an automated bed in the required position. Companion robots, as an assistive technology, are also used in AAL. Finally, with the advent of the IoT (Internet of Things), any physical object at home connected to the Internet (e.g. a light bulb, or a refrigerator) can be considered part of the AAL ICT system's hardware.

With respect to software elements, all AAL systems have basic components for communication and coordination of all the software modules (i.e. sensor and actuator handlers, services, and applications) taking part within the system. This is called middleware. On top of the middleware, basic services are built, for example, a chat service to connect the elderly user, caregivers and family; an alarm service to start emergency processes when required; or monitoring services to continuously gather and track the evolution of variables of interest. Depending on the capabilities of the AALS, it is possible to find pattern recognition services in charge of modeling the user and detecting any anomalous behaviour from the generated patterns (e.g. the user has suffered a fall or has fainted, and, as a consequence, their behavior is not as expected). Also, the AALS may exhibit autonomous behavior, i.e. it might be designed to take the initiative in, hopefully, some perfectly controlled situations. The higher the system level of autonomy, the lower the workload for the caregivers. A sufficiently high level of AAL autonomy can replace the need for the elderly user to have complex interactions with the AALS, something specially important for users that are unfamiliar with technology or who are suffering cognitive deficits. The ICT technology involved in AAL systems must be designed to monitor and assist the human subject 24×7. Thus, an important part of the overall development effort must be oriented to creating friendly systems that are easy to interact with.

3.2   Assisted Healthcare

In response to Moores Law that observes the doubling in the speed of computer hardware every two years, Kurzweil [11] predicts that 2045 will be the year of

---

[2] www.aal-europe.eu.

[3] Thus, it can be said that the term AAL has a European context; it is hardly found in research programs outside Europe, but this is only an issue of terminology.

the Singularity when computers meet or exceed human computational ability. Indeed, the computers' ability to recursively improve themselves can lead to an intelligence explosion, which ultimately affects all aspects of human culture and technology. While the technological singularity remains controversial, the healthcare singularity also appears to attract considerable attention. Due to advances in technology, the translation of medical discovery to practice has improved substantially, from 265 years in 1865 when Lancaster first demonstrated the way to prevent scurvy in the British Empire, to the current 17 years [12,13].

While more is being done to improve in-patient care in the medical sectors by taking advantage of technology, attention should also be paid to out-patients. In-patient care should make the future hospital 'permissive', i.e., the technology should support the widest possible range of clinical practice, patient access to records, and general well-being. Out-patient care involves people who are living at home with medical conditions, in particular the elderly who are in frequent need of taking medications to maintain health. As stated in a recent article [14], new technology like smart pills, a wireless heart monitor and a robotic surgical assistant could radically reshape patient care.

At the beginning of the century the term ubiquitous healthcare was coined. There is increasing support for the idea that healthcare is accessible, not only from the hospital, but at home, in the office, and even in one's automobile. Tiny sensors gather data on almost any physiological characteristic that can be used to diagnose health problems. While much of the literature focuses on ethical challenges ranging from small-scale individual issues of trust and efficacy (privacy, security, accuracy, etc.) [15], to the societal issues of health and longevity gaps related to economic status, technological issues still remain in order to make the living environment more intelligent, more user friendly, and more reliable.

For example, one system, HealthPAL using tiny sensors to gather data, remains one of the simplest devices to operate. It automatically collects data from compatible, off-the-shelf, medical monitors using a smart cable, or wirelessly via Bluetooth, which is currently available in the UK market.

HealthPAL is currently approved for use in conjunction with glucose meters, blood pressure monitors, weight scales, pulse oximeters and pedometers. As a dedicated device for transmitting health data, HealthPAL eliminates the need for a smart phone or computer to transmit and upload health readings. This promotes higher adoptability and compliance for the patient, and removes the opportunity for the misuse or abuse of data plans and equipment that is commonly associated with cell phone and computer health monitoring. However, because of its singular core function of transmitting biometric data, other ambient systems have to be in place to complement and support the intended user's medication taking monitoring task.

3.3 Medication Support

There are a range of systems to support people taking medication. Medication is typically prescribed for a patient by a physician; this prescription is part of a system that is largely human, though the system is often supported by simple electronic databases. The physician, in concert with their records and the patient, makes sure that the patient is not prescribed separate medications that are incompatible.

The basic prescription system has evolved over several centuries. Undoubtedly errors have been found and the system has evolved to cope with most of these.

If, for instance, the medication is prescribed to be taken twice daily for a week, the patient may merely remember to have it at breakfast and dinner from Saturday to the next Friday. They may also make a paper list, or they may set an alarm on their mobile phone to remind them twice a day.

In hospitals and care homes, staff may administer medication, typically keeping a record. Out-patients should adhere to an appropriate medicine taking regime. Specifically, the people in consideration should remember to take necessary medicines at the right time and the right doses. Some people might have different prescriptions from very different clinicians (e.g., dentists and cardiologists); a drug taking support system should be able to discern conflicting medicines and be in the position to inform users the time intervals for taking them or not to take some of them at all. With the proliferation of advanced technologies, the task of taking prescribed medicine can be made easier and safer.

With the advent of an array of ICT technology, many medicine management systems are in place to assist this task and to monitor the progress. In most cases, those systems use a radio-frequency identification (RFID) tag that is usually attached to the medicine product to identify and track the objects based on radio waves [16]. Such tags can be detected and read within a range of several meters. For example, in Addenbrooke's hospital in Cambridge in the UK, by the application of an RFID system to track tagged items via fixed portals and handheld readers, the labour cost has been reduced by half, and drug misuse has been effectively prevented [17]. The only remaining pitfall is that tags are only attached to medicine cases, which does not guarantee that the medicine is taken. For example, a tagged item has been opened. Then the user might proceed to prepare water and then be interrupted by a phone call, resulting in them forgetting to take the medicine. In this case, a video camera based monitoring system might detect the problem.

On the other hand, with regard to assisting drug taking, a drug management system has been proposed to allow users to follow drug schedules as illustrated in Fig. 1. The system features a touch screen interface, bar code scanning facility, and voice and vibration feedback mechanisms to prompt users to take medicine. In addition to communication mechanisms with clinicians about medical treatment and with HIS to refresh needed information, there are mechanisms to provide a memory aid and medicine safety to ensure the effectiveness of self-care at home. Although still in its prototype, the system has shown potential in circumventing a number of issues that are encountered while staying at home alone, especially for elderly or ill people. For example, losing memory, less mobility, and reduced hearing ability all contribute to problems in the solitary home. In parallel, however, people living alone have the advantages of knowing their homes better, familiarity with their living space, and above all being optimistic knowing they are independent and that they can do whatever they like in their own home.

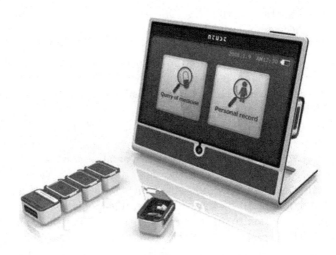

Fig. 1. A drug management system proposed at a MedGudget show [18].

The above system has its pitfalls. For example, communication with hospital HIS poses more challenges than the development of such system itself mainly due to technical compatibilities between different subsystems compounding the main one. In a typical hospital, the HIS in each department are usually installed from different vendors and therefore have their own compatibility issues. A more realistic, simpler system is proposed based on RFID and wireless sensors technique [19]. It employs a fuzzy logic approach to define rules for decision making, sending warning messages at a predicted time of taking medicine. Those predictions are deduced from users' everyday living habits, in particular, the time range when they take their daily meals.

Again, this system cannot assure the intended medicine is taken because a disruption may occur between medicine being taken from an RFID tagged case to the user's mouth. As a result, for example, a relatively simple solution would be a video camera based monitoring system to ensure that the right medicine is indeed taken at the right time with the right dose, which will subsequently lead to the safe taking of prescribed drugs; in some cases, the sequence of drugs plays a crucial role in maintaining a user's health. This system is shown in Fig. 2.

In addition, the system should be able to figure out any conflicts between the medicine a user is going to take, and calculate the safest interval to take them, or to issue a recommendation to see consultants in regard to taking those conflicting medicines.

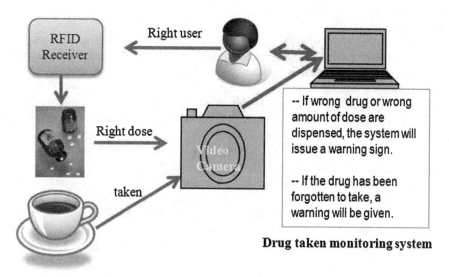

Fig. 2. Proposed system for monitoring medicine taking.

4   On the Horizon

Whilst it is difficult to predict with certainty how popular AAL systems will be in the future and in particular how much of a role they will have in helping with medication intake, the recent uptake of technology at various levels and the interest and investment in the areas here discussed seem to suggest it makes sense to indulge ourselves in a 'what if' exercise. Previous sections have described how automated systems can be deployed at home to provide assistance at various levels and how some of that gadgetry is related to medicine reminders. These medicine reminders have so far been mostly applied to well-structured intake regimes and with medicines that pose less risk to the patient.

If Ambient Intelligence systems driving an AAL application become so powerful that they can work at levels comparable with humans, will they be trusted for the monitoring of more powerful medicines? Will they be able to supervise a patient and advise on medicine intakes which are not rigidly regimented, that is, situations where the decision-making behind taking or not taking medicine is not a certain day and hour but is based on symptoms?

4.1   Potential Problems

An Ambient Intelligence system that is capable to working at the level of humans may be trusted with the task of monitoring the intake of drugs, e.g. pain killers for a person suffering chronic pain. Assessing a patient is often a difficult task even for a fully trained GP, because humans present a rich combination of physical and emotional manifestations. There is also an increased access to information and more people self-medicate. Self-medication by non-medically trained people can sometimes have severe consequences. A GP, based on the account of the patient and other observations and tests, has to navigate their way through a maze of partially overlapping cases discarding some and sometimes considering a number of possible options of equally feasible causes for a condition. Hence a first obstacle for an automated system will be to have access to the same, or at least equally effective, means to gather the data that supports a differential diagnosis. The consequences of getting a diagnosis wrong is that inappropriate medicine or medicine that is taken more often than necessary can have serious untoward consequences. There may also be harmful scenarios that are induced by the patient, for example a hypochondriac may learn how to cheat the system to take more medicine, as they sometimes manage to fool the health system run by humans.

One additional complication here is that humans tend to trust systems that work reasonably well for a while and tend to enjoy the 'peace of mind' reliable automated systems provide [20]. For example, when we turn on our car in the morning we assume it will work, probably because it has been working for the last three years without a problem; experience has led to positive inertial thinking.

4.2 Potential Solutions

Fortunately for humans, we have the skills of hypothesising possible futures and to weigh their pros and cons, a skill which probably developed out of necessity for survival in a hostile planet. Because we can forecast these potential problems, we can also think of ways of avoiding undesirable situations as well as ways of coping with them, which have happened anyway. Probably one of the most reassuring elements of our social life is that there are other humans around us who care about what may happen to us and we are contacted by someone if we have not been in touch for a while. Getting humans in the loop, involving people as part of the process, can be a way to rule out or to ameliorate harmful situations. For example, it can be embedded in the safety of the system that medicine intake systems will need to consult with a number of qualified individuals as external consultants ratifying the decision.

We also suggest a way of progressively getting the human out of the loop. We envisage an ecosystem in which the AAL system starts working with the rest of the elements (i.e. patient, caregivers, family and doctors) silently, just observing, building internal models of behavior and continuously assessing their correctness by comparing their responses with those of the ecosystem's actors. Once the AAL system's internal behavior models deserve enough confidence, it starts suggesting to the actors how to proceed given an event of interest until one day, there is enough evidence for each actor that actions can be delegated to the AAL system.

4.3 Tradeoffs

In a way, the need to consult with external humans (i.e. maintaining the human in the loop) defeats the purpose of AAL systems. The advantages remaining will be that the patient is still allowed to take the medicine at home without the need to go to the hospital and the system of AAL will be 'watered down' to one of telemedicine. However, the benefits of having assistive technology at home should not be ignored because costs are reduced and service quality improved by the patient from the hospital to home.

On the other hand, maintaining facilities with centralised assistive technology has obvious advantages: affordable maintenance costs, easy management of services and controlled decisions when dealing with the patient. Another important issue to consider here that goes against keeping the patient at home is that in such cases the other actors (i.e. humans) may withdraw contact and visits to the vulnerable person under care. This withdrawal can lead to debilitation, and development of new and unforeseen problems.

4.4 Legal Aspects to Consider

Besides the pros and cons of adopting AAL technology in the future, we have to consider also how a possible adoption influences the legal dimension. At the moment, any mention of legal aspects have been intentionally omitted as AAL systems were analysed from a perspective grounded in the present. At the present moment, discussion about the impact of intelligent systems in medicine and healthcare is emerging

However, in the near future, artificial intelligence based systems in general, and those of the ambient intelligence kind in particular, should be subject to legal treatment as a natural consequence of their ever increasing autonomy.

A clear example of a real intelligent system whose autonomy makes itself capable of violating the law is the Google self-driven car, as an example although other manufacturers are also creating their own models. This car is legal on streets in three US states now. It seems obvious that these autonomous vehicles will be seen on our streets in the coming years. But for this to occur, a good balance must be found about who has legal responsibility at the face of an accident: the car (i.e. the manufacturer) or the driver.

The same will occur with autonomous AAL systems with enough responsibility on their decisions to affect people's lives. A suitable trade-off is needed. If most of the legal responsibility is put on the AALS, then companies will be less interested in bringing such potentially problematic products to market. On the other hand, if caregivers, relatives or even the subjects under monitoring are responsible for all actions taken by the AALS, they probably will prefer a not so autonomous but less expensive AAL technology. The right point of equilibrium should be found in the near future. And such a point of equilibrium should be found as a result of a common agreement from experts in many different areas: law, ethics, medicine, philosophy and computer science [21]. This also applies to proto-AGIs beyond AALSs.

5 One Possible Future

There are an infinite number of possible future scenarios, and this section will discuss two scenarios. The first is systems that recommend when to take medication that is taken at irregular intervals, such as pain medication. The second are conversational systems that interact with the user via natural language conversation.

There are a range of medications that are taken irregularly, including at least some times pain medication, weight loss medication, and insulin. Future systems will now be able know to when this irregular medication is needed. This might make use of sophisticated monitoring systems that measure specific physiological properties of the patient, his cognitive state, his diet, and his exercise levels.

In these cases, medicine intake depends on subjective judgment. If the person is in pain, the system may suggest to take medicine, but at a higher dosage than needed. This may lead to unneeded negative side effects.

The future monitoring systems will also be able to make recommendations about information to read about the medicine, and provide links to medical professionals when necessary. The system will of course ensure that ad hoc occasional medicine use does not compromise the existing routine medication, and more importantly, does not cause additional unnecessary unwanted medical conditions.

People have the right to make informed decisions about their own medical treatment. It is crucial that in a wide range of circumstances the person is involved in their own care. They need to be informed about options and risks. The system can point the user to information, and even explain some things. To some extent this can support a physician in this task.

Like other existing Artificial Intelligence systems, conversational systems are domain specific. These 'chatbots' interact with a person via text or even speech. Some simple examples are automated phone operators that give the user options to choose from. More sophisticated systems (e.g. TRAINS [22] or tutorial agents [23]) perform complex domain specific tasks, like scheduling trains, in collaboration with users.

A dialogue system will be able interact with the future user to decide when and which medication to take. It could even be part of a larger AAL conversational system that interacted with the user.

These systems will probably be connected to the Internet, and will be able to learn things from the Internet. They will use sophisticated mechanisms to learn about the user. Current technology such as rule-based systems, Bayesian systems, and neural networks will probably improve. None the less, like now, these systems will be imperfect. Some types of systems are better at some tasks, and other types at others. For example, Bayesian systems are good for learning from a large amount of data, while rule-based systems are good for encoding an expert's knowledge. In recent years, researchers aware of this complementarity have started to use a mix of them, sometimes simultaneously. A solution based in one tool alone will be easier to fix but limited in effectiveness, and one with different parallel tools working at once may be able to cover more situations effectively but more difficult to engineer and fix if something does not go well.

It is unlikely that the medical support system will be able to do a better job than a physician at managing medication and informing the user, but unlike a physician they will be machines. They will be available without fatigue, unlike a physician or nurse. Even if they are more effective than a physician, the person will still need to make some decisions.

When people are unable to make their own decisions, for example infants or people with advanced dementia, a human will continue to have the final authority. The system may try to convince the person, via conversation, but as now, the person with power of attorney will have the final word.

6 Conclusion

AAL is still in its infancy, but is becoming progressively more sophisticated. It will continue to become more complex and will help people in an ever-growing range of tasks. While these systems are useful, like any system, they can have problems. This chapter has used the example domain of systems that assist in medicine taking. It has shown that these systems are in use; that these existing systems have problems; and that these problems can potentially be solved.

Creating an Artificial Intelligence system with an aggregation of methods to make decisions will not be trivial. Possibly more effective solutions lie outside the technical sphere and involve humans.

It is important to find problems before they happen. These problem may have technical solutions, but they may also require a solution from a larger system that involves people. The example of who is legally responsible for an assistant is one issue that must be considered.

Moreover, people will always need to be involved in a range of roles. The example of people having control over their own decisions is one particularly pertinent one. However, people will need to be involved both to empower them, and to make the overall system more effective. The solutions to these problems are also consistent with solutions for possible AGI problems. People want powerful tools, like AGIs and AALSs; however, people still want to be in control. Systems need to have checks both externally and internally to assure that people still retain appropriate control.

AAL systems will aid people more and more in the future. It is important that they are not treated as a panacea, but more as a useful technology that may have flaws. These flaws need to be carefully considered and corrected to give people the most effective assistance.

Acknowledgements. This research has been partially supported by Ministerio de Economía y Competitividad of the Spanish Goverment through the project TIN2011-28335-C02-02. This work also formed part of WIDTH project that was funded by EU FP7 under Marie Curie scheme (2011–2014).

References

1. Tenner, E.: Why things bite back: technology and the revenge of unintended consequences. Vintage (1997)
2. Smolensky, P.: Connectionist AI, symbolic AI, and the brain. Artif. Intell. Rev. **1**, 95–109 (1987)
3. Shi, Z.: Advanced Artificial Intelligence. World Scientific (2011)
4. Cook, D., Augusto, J., Jakkula, V.: Ambient intelligence: technologies, applications, and opportunities. Pervasive Mob. Comput. **5**(4), 277–298 (2009)

5. Bringsjord, S.: Belief in the singularity is logically brittle. J. Conscious. Stud. **19**(7), 14 (2012)
6. Sotala, K., Yampolskiy, R.: Responses to catastrophic AGI risk: a survey. Physica Scripta **90**(1), 018001 (2015)
7. Armstrong, S., Sandberg, A., Bostrom, N.: Thinking inside the box: controlling and using an oracle AI. Mind. Mach. **22**(4), 299–324 (2012)
8. Wallach, W., Allen, C., Smit, I.: Machine morality: bottom-up and top-down approaches for modelling human moral faculties. AI Soc. **22**(4), 565–582 (2008)
9. Dooley, J., Callaghan, V., Hagras, H., Gardner, M., Ghanbaria, M., AlGhazzawi, D.: The intelligent classroom: beyond four walls. In: Proceedings of the Intelligent Campus Workshop (IC 2011) held at the 7th IEEE Intelligent Environments Conference (IE 2011), Nottingham (2011)
10. Augusto, J., Huch, M., Kameas, A., Maitland, J., McCullagh, P., Roberts, J., Sixsmith, A., Wichert, R.: Handbook on Ambient Assisted Living - Technology for Healthcare, Rehabilitation and Well-being. IOS Press (2012)
11. Kurzweil, R.: The Signulairty is Near: When Humans Transcend Biology. Penguin Group, New York (2005)
12. Balas, E.: Information systems can prevent errors and improve quality. J. Am. Med. Inform. Assoc. **8**, 398–399 (2001)
13. Gillam, M., Feied, C., Handler, J., Moody, E., Shneigerman, B., Plaisant, C., Smith, M., Dickason, J.: The healthcare singularity and the age of semantic medicine, the fourth paradigm: data-intensive scientific discovery, pp. 57–64. Microsoft Research (2009)
14. Whelan, C.: The doctor is out, but new patient monitoring and robotics technology is in. Sci. Am. (2010). http://www.scientificamerican.com/article/patient-monitoring-tech/. Accessed November 2015
15. Brown, I., Adoms, A.: The ethical challenges of ubiquitous healthcare. Int. Rev. Inf. Ethics **8**, 53–60 (2010)
16. Jeong, D., Kim, Y., In, H.: New RFID system architectures supporting situation. awareness under ubiquitous environments. J. Comput. Sci. **1**(2), 114–120 (2005)
17. Swedberg, C.: RFID boosts medical equipment usage at U.K. hospital. RFID J. (2013). http://www.rfidjournal.com/articles/view?10916. Accessed November 2015
18. MedGudget: Drug management system (2013)
19. Yamamoto, Y., Huang, R., Ma, J.: Medicine management and medicine taking assistance system for supporting elderly care at home. In: Aware Computing (ISAC) (2010)
20. Augusto, J., McCullagh, P., Augusto-Walkden, J.: Living without a safety net in an intelligent environment. ICST Transactions on Ambient Systems **1**(1) (2011)
21. Collste, G., Duquenoy, P., George, C., Hedstrm, K., Kimppa, K., Mordini, E.: Ict in medicine and health care: assessing social, ethical and legal issues. In: Berleur, J., Nurminen, M., Impagliazzo, J. (eds.) Social Informatics: An Information Society for all? In Remembrance of Rob Kling. IFIP International Federation for Information Processing, vol. 223, pp. 297–308. Springer, US (2006)
22. Allen, J., Schubert, L., Ferguson, G., Heeman, P., Hwang, C., Kato, T., Light, M., Martin, N., Miller, B., Poesio, M., Traum, D.: The trains project: a case study in building a conversational planning agent. J. Exp. Theor. AI **7**, 7–48 (1995)
23. VanLehn, K., Graesser, A., TannerJackson, G., Jordan, P., Olney, A., Rose, C.: When are tutorial dialogues more effective than reading. Cogn. Sci. **31**(1), 3–62 (2007)

Ambient Assisted Living

Ambient Technology to Support Elderly People in Outdoor Risk Situations

Rami Yared$^{(\boxtimes)}$, Hady Khaddaj Mallat, and Bessam Abdulrazak

Université de Sherbrooke, 2500, boul. de l'Université, Sherbrooke, QC, Canada
{rami.yared, Hady.Khaddaj.Mallat,
bessam.abdulrazak}@usherbrooke.ca

Abstract. Elderly people are subjected to several safety issues while performing Activities of Daily Living. On the other hand, Assistive technology is a promising solution to enhance safety of elderly people, and consequently improve their quality of life and independent living. We present in this paper a review of the major risks affecting elderly people in outdoor environment and the related assistive technology.

Keywords: Risk · M-Health · Mobile · Wearable device · Assistive technology · Elderly people · Outdoor · Activities of daily living

1 Introduction

Elderly people face varieties of risks while performing Activities of Daily Living (ADL), due to physical, sensorial and cognitive decline. This situation requires high attention because the number of elderly people is increasing constantly all over the world. The numbers are particularly critical in the developed countries, since the advance in healthcare systems has enabled longer life. In Canada, the proportion of elderly people aged 65 years or over will represent between 23 % and 25 % of the population by 2036, and between 24 % and 28 % by 2061 [13, 52]. In Japan, the population of 65 year-old was about 25.1 % of the total population in 2013, and will be 40 % in 2050, which is the highest ratio of aging population in the world [87] In the United States, the number of elderly people is also on the rise: in 2010, there were 40.3 million people aged 65 and above, comprising 13 % of the overall population. This proportion is 12 times higher than it was in 1900, when this group constituted only 4.1 % of the population. By 2050, projections indicate the population over 65 will comprise 20.9 % of the population in the United States [48]. In Europe, by 2025 more than 20 % of population will be 65 or over, with a particularly rapid increase in the number of elderly people over 80 s. In the United States, 40 % of women and 19 % of men aged 65 years and older, live alone and do not have anyone in the home to assist with activities of daily living, provide care when they are sick, or to assist with home maintenance [37]. Therefore, researchers are paying a special attention toward condition of elderly people including work on: understanding the population, their needs, challenges faced, and risks in ADL.

© Springer International Publishing Switzerland 2015
M. Helfert et al. (Eds.): ICT4AgeingWell 2015, CCIS 578, pp. 35–56, 2015.
DOI: 10.1007/978-3-319-27695-3_3

Several factors prevent elderly people from being active including physical, psychological and social barriers [9, 89]. Elderly people become less active and more prone to social isolation and loneliness, which complicate their health situation and cause premature mortality [96]. On the other hand, participation in activities has promising benefits at physical, sociological and psychological levels [82]. This participation can result in lower risk of dementia and improves well-being [54]. Moreover, physical activity slows down the progression of diseases, and it is in general a promoter of health. Increasing participation in social activities improves cognitive abilities for elderly people [42], and consequently leads to a higher Quality of Life (QoL).

The interventions to reduce the consequences of risks affecting elderly people can be classified in two categories: human and technological interventions. The human intervention includes health and social assistance, provided by caregivers or relatives accompanying elderly people. This approach may have negative impacts on elderly people including emotional impact (e.g., since it reduces the privacy space of elderly people) and economic impact (e.g., it is often associated with a cost to the person, family or the health system). On the other hand, the recent advances in ICT (e.g., m-health, pervasive technologies (based on context awareness [2], Internet of Things, cloud computing, and sensor networks) enabled the creation of new categories of solutions that may assist elderly people in ADL. Two common terms are interchangeably used in the literature to identify technology to assist elderly people: Assistive Technology (**AT**) and Gerontechnology.

The most frequent risks in outdoor environment are: fall, wandering, health issues, traffic accidents, fatigue, abuse, crime, and psychological related risks. (We mean by outdoor environment any environment outside home, including open-air areas). The most addressed risks by ICT are fall, wandering, and health issues [39]. Therefore, we mainly review these major risks, and discuss related assistive technology in this paper. To describe the progress made in this domain, we searched and matched real work and existing technology for each risk. Our goal is to better understand the recent progress in assistive technology. To the best of our knowledge, this paper is the first review on assistive technology related to risks faced by elderly people in outdoor ADL.

This paper is organized as follows. After this introduction, Sect. 2 introduces the methodology followed in our research. Section 3 describes the major risks that elderly people face in outdoor environment. Section 4 presents Assistive Technology and m-health systems that help elderly people in risk situations. In this section, we mainly focus on reviewing the assistive technologies that have been developed to provide assistance for the three major risks. We also introduce our framework of existing assistive technology. Finally, Sect. 5 concludes the paper and discusses ongoing and future directions.

2 Methodology

Our goal is to provide a review on the major risks affecting elderly people in outdoor environment as well as on technology that may help them, rather than a systematic review. We present in this section the methodology we used to identify the major risks, and to review the existing research on assistive technology for these risks. Our methodology is based on the literature identified through a search on the following databases: *PubMed, ScienceDirect, IEEE Xplore* and *Google Scholar*. These are the main databases that catalogue the research on risk factors faced by elderly people in outdoor ADL and the related assistive technology.

- We searched PubMed for the following terms: "risk factor," "danger situation," "hazard," "emergency," "outdoor," "barrier" and "frailness." The choice of these terms in PubMed is motivated by the fact that this database is specialized in human/medical factors.
- The ScienceDirect, Google Scholar, and IEEE Xplore databases were searched for combinations of the terms "elderly people," "assistive technology," "teleassistance," "mobile health," "pervasive healthcare" and the terms listed above. The choice of these terms and databases is motivated by the fact that these databases are more technology related.

Based on reading of the abstracts retrieved from databases, we identified articles that describe risks and hazards that affect elderly people. We also identified potential assistive technology that may support elderly people in these risk situations.

We disregarded in our study articles that discuss research related to elderly people in other contexts (e.g., studies on chronic diseases, disabilities or other minor risks with no existing related assistive technology). For each article in the resulting set, along with other articles cited in the resulting article set, we identified how major risks affect elderly people in their ADL. We also extracted devices systems or applications that may assist elderly people facing such risks, and identified the three main addressed risks. We then iteratively clustered the risks and assistive technology until we arrived at the ˙categorization described in this paper, as well as our framework for existing assistive technology related to outdoor risks.

3 Major Risks in Outdoor Environment

Various hazards cause risks for elderly people in outdoor environments. We identified the three major risks addressed in the literature as: fall, wandering and health issues. Other risks may include: traffic accidents, fatigue, dehydration, environmental factors (e.g., ambient temperature, sunlight overexposure), mistreatment, abuse, crime, and suicide. The three risks (and others) may precipitate the following common consequences:

- **Physical:** imply injury and impairments.
- **Psychological:** include fear of further hazards and risks, distress, and embarrassment.
- **Social**: imply loss of independence, mobility and social ties, as well as high probability to move into residential/healthcare facilities.
- **Financial and Medical:** include higher cost and medical efforts linked to the handling of the risk situation. This burden can be on personal financial, relative and health systems.

- **Governmental and Communitarians:** imply hospital admissions (e.g. number of beds) and health insurance cost.

These undesirable risk consequences affect elderly people widely. Therefore, research and industry present various practical solutions to detect, prevent, assist in risk situation, and to alleviate the consequences.

Risk situation may have numerous causes and factors. Inspired from World Health Organization (WHO) International Classification of Functioning disability and health [92], we can highlight three major factors: personal, health and environmental.

- **Personal Factors** may include age, sex, education level, social involvement and previous accidents (risk faced situations).
- **Health Factors** include medical/genetic problems such as visual and cognitive impairment, reduced sensation, and use of medications.
- **Environmental Factors** comprise all the contextual information on the visited environments, including hygiene, pollution and weather condition, obstacles, lighting level, floor leveling and walking surfaces.

Assistive technology is part of the "Environmental factors" that can be used to handle risks. Following, we discuss each of the three major risks separately.

3.1 Fall

Fall can be considered as the possibility of an involuntary and sudden change in position, causing an individual landing at a lower level such as the floor, the ground, or an object, with or without injury [22].

Fall is the most common and frequent risk that elderly people face in outdoor ADL. In fact, a Canadian study revealed that 65 % of falls among elderly people occurred outdoors, while they are walking on a familiar route [22].

Personal factors that may cause fall include mainly age and previous falls. Health factors include chronic medical problems such as, reduced sensation, muscular weakness, and diseases as stroke. Environmental factors comprise poor lighting, sliding floor and slippery surfaces [22, 29, 38]. In addition to the common consequences presented above, psychological consequences include extreme fear of further falls [29] and social consequences as limited outdoor activities.

3.2 Wandering and Disorientation

Wandering can be considered as a psychomotor instability that leads elderly people to move toward unspecified destination. Disorientation is referred to as getting lost because of missing referential points [31]. Wandering is more frequent for elderly people because of memory impairment, particularly those who have dementia or Alzheimer disease [67, 95]. Around 35.6 million people live with dementia throughout the world (According to the WHO). Wandering concerns 11 % of independent people and 28 % of those who need occasional help [12]. Wandering and disorientation may lead elderly people to dangerous situations while performing outdoor activities. In situations where elderly people are disoriented or lost, they become more frightened [26], and subject to abuse [33] (Sect. 3.6). In addition, wandering has social and psychological consequences including fidgety of elderly people and anxiety of relative/family, as well as high risks of losing independence and transferring to special facilities to ensure safety.

3.3 Health Issues

Health issue is defined as the state in which the person is unable to function normally without pain. Health issues are often defined as physiological malfunctioning and impairment [15]. Health issues are unwelcome accompaniments to advancing age for the majority of elderly people. Most elderly people suffer from a variety of symptoms and at least one chronic disease [15]. The most known diseases when aging are the cardiovascular system disease (e.g., heart attack), the respiratory system diseases (e.g., Bronchitis), diabetes mellitus, hypothermia, hypertension, mental problems (e.g., Alzheimer and Parkinson's diseases) [36, 49]. In Europe, cardiovascular diseases cause 45 % of deaths among people aged 75 years or younger [60]. These medical conditions are highly prevalent among elderly people, and may affect them severely till causing death. The improvement of healthcare systems around the world has enabled elderly people to live longer. However, this phenomenon is associated with an extreme burden on healthcare system budgets and shortage in medical specialized caregivers [35].

Medications compliance or adherence refers to the extent to which a patient accurately follows a medical or healthcare plan [61]. Elderly people are among those most vulnerable to medication adherence, and compliance due to memory impairments [80]. In addition, elderly people use more prescription and over-the-counter medications more than other age groups [73]. Elderly patients use prescription medications approximately three times as frequently as the general population. Approximately 25 % of elderly people use prescription psychoactive medications that have a potential to be misused [76]. Therefore, non-adherence to medication, and drug misuse constitute a high risk for elderly people.

3.4 Traffic Accidents Risk

Elderly people may face traffic accidents while outdoor ADL. According to [5], the two most common situations arrive on walking or driving. The first one "walking" mainly occurs when elderly people need to cross a road and fail to estimate the distance of an approaching vehicle. In Canada between 2000 and 2004, one third of the pedestrians that died in motor vehicle accidents were elderly people. They are considered to be in higher risk than the rest of the population [70]. The second one "driving" takes place when elderly people drive and provoke accidents. It mainly occurs in road intersections, and when they fail to monitor the surrounding environment (e.g., notice street signs). Both situations derive from the health state of elderly people, since they experience a decrease in balance, vision, and hearing, muscle mass, bone mass and cognitive impairments which make them more vulnerable [5]. In addition, long duration of driving is a significant cause of fatigue-related accidents on major roadways.

Transportation safety can be compromised due to the fatigue caused by extended periods of driving which impairs elderly people alertness and performance [85].

3.5 Fatigue Risk

Fatigue is an overwhelming sense of tiredness, lack of energy and a feeling of exhaustion, associated with impaired physical and/or cognitive functioning [75]. Fatigue is a commonly reported risk in elderly people, which has been associated with sedentary lifestyle, poor functional performance and higher levels of disability. Estimations show that up to 50 % of elderly people suffer from mild fatigue [90]. Multiple biological and psychosocial factors may influence fatigue risk. Biological mechanisms include changes in skeletal muscle function, cardiovascular impairment, anemia, dehydration and electrolyte disorders, inflammatory mediators, and nutritional deficiencies. Psychosocial factors include depression, and pain [57]. Reduced muscle function may also contribute to feelings of fatigue when performing mobility-related tasks, such as walking and climbing stairs. Mobility-related fatigue was defined as "a subjective feeling of fatigue in mobility tasks required for independent community living" [51]. Fatigue risk is a strong predictor of functional limitations, disability, mortality, and other adverse outcomes in elderly populations, between men and women, and in different geographic areas [7]. Fatigue risk may reduce mobility-related ADL and lead to a poor quality of life for elderly people [28]. Fatigue risk also limits elderly people driving possibilities (Sect. 3.4).

3.6 Mistreatment, Abuse and Criminal Actions

Elderly mistreatment encompasses: physical, sexual, or psychological abuse, financial and material exploitation, and neglect. The perpetrators could be both family members and acquaintances. The mistreatment could be involuntary or unintentional acts (e.g., physical abuse by a cognitively impaired spouse) [47]. The mistreatment is considered as a risk due to the high vulnerability of elderly people. Other crimes commit against elderly people may include conventional crimes such as robbery, theft, fraud, rape, and murder. It is estimated that approximately 4/1000 elderly people experience nonfatal violent crimes [41]. The impact of victimization is increased due to the aging associated declines [11]. Furthermore, elderly people feel frightened from being a victim of crimes when they perform outdoor ADL. This fear among elderly people is real and pervasive, resulting an adversely impacts to their quality of life.

3.7 Psychological Related Risks

Elderly people usually suffer from several psychological issues, including depression and stress due to loneliness, isolation, and cognitive decline. Insomnia is considered as a risk factor for depression. Depression results in persistent bad mood and lack of interest in pursuing daily life. Depression may have serious and sometimes long-term consequences that can affect every aspect of life [66]. The lack of physical and social activities can lead elderly people to depression, increase their feeling of loneliness. Furthermore, stress may also have health consequences and adversely affect the immune, cardiovascular, and central nervous systems. Stress may result in serious health conditions including anxiety, insomnia, muscle pain, high blood pressure and a weakened immune system [10]. These psychological issues may lead elderly people to suicide risk.

Protective factors include higher education and engagement in activities, and religious or spiritual involvement [69]. Preventive interventions include education and group support [93]. Interventions to prevent and reduce suicide risk, are based on handling the complications of depression, abuse, sleep disturbances, pain, and disability in elderly people [14, 16]. In addition, enhancing physical prosperity may lead to improved psychological situation and it is generally accepted that physical activity may have positive effects on mood [81].

4 Assistive Technologies for Major Outdoor Risks

Elderly people are strongly concerned by outdoor risks. Therefore, elderly people are often forced to move to a nursing home or healthcare facility. Urgent intervention is required to prevent or reduce risks. A possible solution is an accompanying caregiver or a family member. However, this solution is not practical due to independency issues. In addition, it has several drawbacks such as high cost and elderly people has to accept the idea of being not completely autonomous. These factors negatively affect the moral situation of elderly people and consequently complicate the cognitive deficiencies recovery [77]. Therefore, assistive technology is an interesting alternative to enhance safety of elderly people in outdoor environments.

Embedding artificial intelligence in ICT, context-awareness approaches, and connecting heterogeneous devices have a wide potential of utilization in different outdoor situations [27, 71].

The architecture of existing assistive technology systems can be viewed as follows.

- Sensor devices (e.g., Global Positioning System (GPS), RFID, accelerometer, bio-sensors) allow acquisition of contextual data;
- Various mobile and wearable computing devices (e.g., personal computers, smart phones, tablets) facilitate context collection, aggregation and processing;
- Applying artificial intelligence techniques allow quantification and detection of human behavior;
- Approaches for positioning, monitoring, orientation, navigation, and communication enable continuous outdoor assistance of elderly people.

The progress of assistive technology is continuous until establishing digital smart environments that are sensitive, adaptive, and responsive to human needs, habits, gestures, and emotions [6]. Advances in the development of technologies have the potential to extend the assistance from indoor (e.g., home, office, care facility) to outdoor, and provide a continuum of assistance in an Open Smart Environment [2, 3]. Building an open smart environment to assist elderly people outdoor requires the integration of computational methodologies (Algorithms) and ambient intelligence [27]. There are three main areas of research in this domain.

(1) Monitoring and sensing: design and develop technology for remote monitoring and sensing, in order to identify instantly and accurately the contextual environmental changes, through the use of sensors, mobile and software tools for automated data collection and their analysis.
(2) Risk detection: design and develop technology for early detection of hazards, risks and accidents, to trigger an emergency intervention.
(3) Intervention: design and develop tools for: *(i)* localization of an elderly people; *(ii)* coordination and planning of the intervention; *(iii)* usable and useful human machine interaction for better intervention.

Researchers have more focused on developing assistive technology for home assistance (indoor) [58] in comparison with outdoor Assistive Technology. The technical limitations of work on outdoor Assistive Technology are due to:

- The heterogeneity of contextual information acquired via sensors.
- The lack of standards, and the heterogeneity of the semantics, syntax, languages and protocols used by the various providers in outdoor environments.
- The highly changing and in some cases unstable environmental conditions (e.g., availability of wireless communication, accessibility of network services).
- The complexity of managing user mobility.
- The complexity of building applications that handle the above items.

Outdoor assistive technologies are mainly based on wearable devices to manage risks (such as sensors embedded in clothes, watches, belts, and smartphones). Several of the existing solutions are hardware custom based, which increase the cost of development and pricing, as consequences limits the solvability of their market. The companies that commercialize devices also provide developers with programming IDEs that facilitate building applications with different aims. The wave of smart devices has enabled reducing the cost of developing applications significantly. Researchers focus more on application rather than hardware. As consequences, numerous m-health and outdoor assistive technologies have been developed for the major mobile platforms (e.g., iOS, Android, Blackberry) [40]. Assisting elderly people outdoor can be performed following a specific request from user or an automatic detection of a situation. The specific request can be an emergency call triggered by user with the help of a simple mobile interface (e.g., panic button) [4, 30]. The framework for handling risks contains multiple phases including data acquisition by monitoring and sensing, data processing,

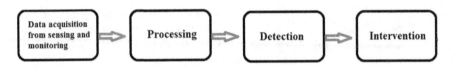

Fig. 1. Schema of assistive technology framework.

detection of the risk and interventions by calling emergency center or caregivers (Fig. 1).

Following we discuss in details the assistive technologies linked to the three major risks (fall, wandering, and health issues) from the point of view of existing research work on assistive technology, how these technologies assist elderly people, and how technology improves their quality of life. We also introduce our framework for handling risks. In addition, we briefly discuss the existing assistive technology for other risks such as traffic accidents, fatigue, crime, and psychological related risks. Due to the lack of existing assistive technologies for those risks, we limit the associated section to a discussion on the functioning principles and to an introduction of representative examples.

4.1 Assistive Technology for Fall Risk

Diverse methods can be used to detect fall. According to Mubashir and Yu [56, 97], a fall can be detected by three main techniques, through the use of wearable devices, ambient devices and vision-based devices (i.e. camera). Therefore, the use of this technology can detect falls whether they happen in outdoor or indoor environments. However, in assistive technology for outdoor environment, fall detection is mainly performed through the use of wearable devices, such as smartphones and sensors. These mobile devices can also help to create support from caregivers to help elderly people in the best delay. This can be done by using several methods and algorithms. The goal is to select, and then to communicate with the best available caregivers around the injured person. An exhaustive review for body worn sensors to detect falls has been made by Schwickert et al. [74]. The authors listed, gathered and discussed a

Table 1. Examples of existing assistive technology (AT) for fall risk.

App. & accelerometer sensor	Smartphone-based fall detection applications (app) that monitor the movements of user, recognize a fall, and automatically send a request for help.	iFall [78]
		MyVigi [12]
		PerfallD [21]
	The applications are based on smartphone embedded sensors (e.g. three axial accelerometer, motion).	E-FallD [17]
		[1]
	An adaptive threshold algorithm is used to distinguish fall. In case of fall, prerecorded emergency contacts (e.g., relative, caregiver) are contacted by phone call, SMS and email.	FallAlarm [98]
Body sensor network	Wearable motion detection device using tri-axial accelerometer or/and Gyroscopes to detect and predict falls.	Accurate, Fast Fall Detection [44]
		[86]
Watch-worn based on sensor	The detector is easy to wear and offers the full functionality of a small transportable wireless alarm system.	SPEEDY [23]
Wearable camera	An activity classification system using wearable cameras is used to detect falls. Since user wears the camera, monitoring is not limited to confined areas. It extends to wherever user may go (indoor and outdoor)	[62]

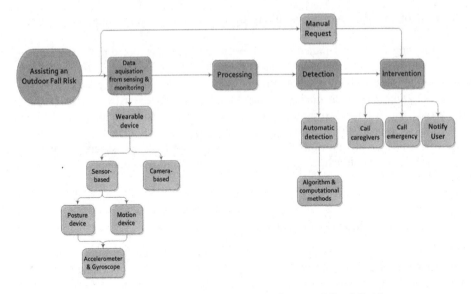

Fig. 2. Schema of assistive technology framework for fall risk.

representative published work on fall and body-worn sensors. Examples of existing assistive technology that address fall risk are illustrated in Table 1. We depict in Fig. 2 the logic of handling fall risk using assistive technology.

The data acquisition from wearable devices, such as accelerometer or camera, represents the first phase. After that, this data is analyzed and processed to detect a fall risk. The detection of fall is obtained from different algorithms and computational methods as many approaches. The last phase is the intervention of caregivers to assist injured person in the best delay. For example, calling and notifying an emergency call center or a family member.

4.2 Assistive Technology for Wandering Risk

Advances in sensing, monitoring, communication and computing techniques enable safe walking and accurate navigation. Existing solutions for wandering detection are mainly based on GPS. According to Lin et al. [46], there are three types of key techniques that were applied in the existing work to assist elderly people in case of wandering in outdoor environment: event monitoring, trajectory tracking, and localization combined with Geo-fence technique.

(1) Event monitoring technique: is to determine a wandering behavior based on activity monitoring. Through the analysis of these events, we may detect a wandering behavior in case of rhythmical repetition.

(2) Trajectory tracking technique: detects wandering risk using the trajectory tracking technique, while motion trajectories differ from trajectories patterns that the elderly people are supposed to take.

(3) Localization combined with Geo-fence technique: consists on user localization in outdoor environment and analyzes this location to detect any deviations or boundary transgressions.

Table 2. Examples of existing assistive technology (AT) for wandering risk.

Tech.	Assistive Technology	Ref
App, GPS & GIS	**GPS based systems** to detect wandering risk. These systems enable caregiver (or family members / volunteers) to register safe zones for user. If the user moves outside the safe zones for a predetermined time, the system infers wandering situation using various algorithms (e.g., Bayesian). These systems may have various features including: navigate user home after detecting a wandering risk, send notifications to caregiver containing user-location (by phone call, SMS and/or email), establishes a line of communication between user and caregiver, as well as a web site with real-time localization map. These systems can be: • Based on worn GPS sensor (e.g., on Shoes, belt, watch): These systems are hardware custom based. The worn part is mainly composed of a GPS sensor and signal transmission modules to transfer the position coordinates to a central monitoring station. The central monitoring station is in charge of processing the wandering risk (e.g., **GPS-Shoes**). • Based on a GPS sensor integrated in a smart device (e.g., smartphone, smart glasses, and smart watch): In this case, the devices have processing resources and the risk is often processed/detected by an app (e.g., **iWander** and **MyVigi**).	[79] [12] [45] [63]
App & camera	**DejaView** is a camera-based system designed to aid recall of daily activities, plans, people, places, and objects. It senses (using the camera) the user's surroundings and inferring context. The system then unobtrusively cues users with relevant information, helping them orientate themselves and aiding both their prospective and retrospective memory.	[24]
App, Camera & worn laser device	**Camera based systems** to remotely guide users. The systems provide navigation aid in complex and unknown areas. These systems are often composed of camera, compass and GPS. The remote center (caregiver location) can manually or automatically interpret user-data to infer the user status. In case of assistance need, the caregiver can remotely access the scene of the user using the user worn camera. These systems also enable caregiver to guide/direct the user by speech or by laser-projected arrows.	[84] [94]

Examples of existing technological solutions to handle wandering risk are illustrated in Table 2. Our framework of assistive technology for outdoor wandering risk has four phases (Fig. 3): data acquisition from wearable devices, data processing, detection of the wandering risk and the intervention to assist elderly people such as making an emergency call or a caregiver call.

4.3   Assistive Technology for Health Issues (M-Health)

The adoption of mobile and wireless technologies in healthcare improves health services. Providing healthcare services in outdoor environments is mainly performed by m-health technology. M-Health (i.e., Mobile Health) is a domain aims at improving the health of patients through mobile and wireless devices, networks, servers, and software applications. The World Health Organization (WHO) defines m-health as: "*Medical and*

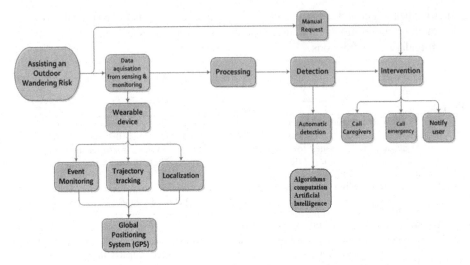

Fig. 3. Schema of assistive technology framework for wandering risk.

public health practice supported by mobile devices, such as mobile phones, patient monitoring devices, personal digital assistants, and other wireless devices. M-Health involves the use and capitalization on a mobile phone's core utility of voice and short messaging service as well as more complex functionalities." m-health covers a large spectrum of applications (e.g., health monitoring and diagnostics, well-being, medication adherence/compliance, health education, and caregiver support). Applications for medication adherence/compliance support patients to be compliant with their designated treatment plan with features including interactive medication and appointment reminders along with patient education [53]. Assistive Technology for medication compliance is based on pervasive automatic reminders for medication use. WOT is a system for medication adherence using an ingestible electronic sensor attached to a tablet. After ingestion, the sensor separates from the medication, activated by gastric fluid, and communicates with the monitor that is worn on the user's torso. The information stored in the monitor is sent wirelessly using Bluetooth to a mobile phone [25].

We focus in this subsection on m-health applications that are related to the category of health monitoring and diagnostics. M-health is mainly performed by the help of wireless technology, sensors and wearable devices (often named WBSN: Wearable Body Sensor Network). The sensor network is made of wearable biosensors and actuators that are interconnected to gather the patient's functional and contextual parameters. These sensors can vary depending on the type of the collected data, e.g., Electrocardiography (ECG), Electroencephalography (EEG), Pulse Oximeter Oxygen Saturation (SpO2), heart and respiration rates, blood pressure, glucose level, body temperature, and spatial location. In addition, these WBSN systems also consist of a mobile unit that implements applications with the use of built-in sensors (e.g., camera, GPS, and accelerometers). These mobile units connect with the body sensor network forming a system together. Furthermore, using wireless technology and wearable devices allow notifying elderly people about their health status, and also alert caregivers and people nearby of emergency situations. In presence of shortage of healthcare experts, m-health plays an important role. Just a simple example on how m-health can help facing the shortage of an expert caregiver: the task of a nurse that monitors the health status of an elderly person each day can be alleviated by using a body sensor network system.

M-health applications related to health monitoring and diagnostics can be categorized in four categories (may overlap) according to the information flow and the frequency of information flow between patients and caregivers [18].

(1) **Self-healthcare Management:** This category focuses on the autonomy, engagement and self-confidence of patients, without the need for involvement of an external caregiver in the delivery of m-health services.

(2) **Assisted Solutions:** This category relies on the assistance of a contact person or a caregiver in emergency situations, and the data is transferred to this assistant person in particular the location of the patient who needs help.

(3) **Supervised Healthcare:** This category comprises a monitoring system that mainly involves a remote database where the collected health related data is periodically sent and stored. The advantage this category is that it enables caregivers to remotely access and manage the current and past data of patients, recorded on the medical database.

(4) **Continuous Monitoring:** This category includes all the functionalities described in the previous categories, with the collected data sent continuously to caregivers. This category is characterized by more sophisticated data analysis and interventions than the previous categories.

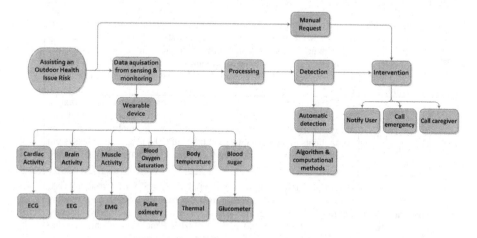

Fig. 4. Schema of m-health framework.

Table 3 depicts well-known existing m-health systems designed to assist elderly people in diverse health issues, including cardiovascular, diabetes, hypertension, and Parkinson diseases.

Our framework for m-health is illustrated in Fig. 4.

Table 3. Examples of m-health solutions.

Health issues	Tech.	Functionality of the system	Ref.
Cardiovascular	Custom mobile health monitoring unit & wearable ECG sensors	A custom mobile health monitoring system using WBSN. The system is based on ECG connected to a network hub or a 3G phone for cardiac arrhythmias detection. The used real-time ambulatory ECG detection algorithm enables diagnosis for cardiac arrhythmia events. In case of emergency, it establishes a direct interaction between users and service providers.	[43]
	WBSN, Wearable ECG & Android app.	A mobile health monitoring system using WBSN and Android phone. The system operates similarly to the previous one. The Android phone (in the case of this system) processes the data and detects abnormal situation (alarm). The phone also forwards the alarm (with ECG data) to a cloud Alarm Server, which pushes the messages to doctors' phone.	[34]
Cardiac & Hypertension	WBSN & Android app.	iCare is a mobile health monitoring system using WBSN and smart phone. Similarly to the previous systems, this one monitors the health status (Cardiac & Hypertension) of elderly people and provides tailored services for each person based on personal health condition. When detecting an emergency, the smart phone automatically alert pre-assigned people (who could be a family member or a friend) and call an emergency center.	[50]
Diabetes	Mobile app. & peripheral sensors	A mobile phone application designed for self-care management of people with Diabetes Mellitus type 1. The system enables to keep notes of personal data (e.g., pre-measured glucose levels and blood pressure, food and drink intake, physical activity). In case of feeling unwell or an emergency, user can press a button to transmit immediately his/her position with the personal data to both an emergency call center and an attendant physician.	[55]
Respiratory	WBSN (Wristband sensors and pulse-oxymeter) & Smartphone app.	SweetAge system is WBSN base on wristband sensors and pulse-oxymeter connection to a smartphone via Bluetooth. It enables to tele-monitor vital signs (i.e., oxygen saturation, heart rate, near-body temperature). The system displays an alert in case of abnormal respiratory situation (a measurement is outside the predefined range). The system instructs users to contact their health care providers in case of need.	[65]
Parkinson	On-body acceleration sensors	A WBSN composed of on-body acceleration sensors to assist people with Parkinson's disease. The system measures user movement and automatically detects Freezing Of Gait (FOG) by analyzing frequency components inherent in movement. When FOG is detected, the system generates a rhythmic auditory signal to stimulate user to resume walking.	[8]
General	Mobile app. (& bracelet in the future).	iHELP is a mobile application mainly designed for heart attack risk, but could be extended to other risks. It offers a quick and easy sending of multiple SOS alarm messages to family members, friends, professional rescuers and all users of iHELP mobile application within a radius of 300 meters (The radius can be configured).	[60]
	WBSN & mobile app.	PEACH integrates various bio-sensors in a WBSN (including blood pressure sensors, respiration sensors, and skin conductivity sensors) to detect alterations of physical conditions and dangerous health situations. It assists user by quickly create an ad hoc rescue groups of nearby volunteers.	[83]

4.4   Assistive Technologies for Other Risks in Outdoor Environment

In this subsection, we briefly discuss assistive technology developed to help elderly people in other risk situations. (i.e., traffic accidents, fatigue, crime, and psychological related risks). We also cite a representative example of assistive technology for each risk.

4.4.1   AT for Traffic Accidents

For the first category (Driving), there are technological facilities for driving car and improving the comfort of elderly people while driving. An example of representative solutions can be: adjustable power seats, adjustable foot pedals, large wide-angle mirrors and large rear windows aid visibility, and can work with a rear backup camera, active parallel-park assistance, and front and rear parking sensors to help elderly drivers maneuver their vehicles without engaging in too much of the upper-body twisting and turning that can be painful for those with stiffness in the neck or shoulders [19]. The fatigue related solutions are addressed in the next subsection (AT for fatigue risk).

For the second category (walking), the existing assistive applications are based on the same technology designed to assist elderly people in fall risk (Sect. 4.1), or in emergency situations [78].

4.4.2   AT for Fatigue Risk

Technology advances allow the detection of fatigue, mainly through monitoring performance via surface electromyography (sEMG) systems. These systems allow to capture EMG signals using a wearable device, recognize muscular fatigue, and provide a feedback to user. As a representative example, Pioggia et al. developed a system that provides an early detection of excessive fatigue and activity abnormalities minimizing the risk [68].

For fatigue while driving, the methods of fatigue detection mainly focused on measurements of the driver's state, driver performance and the combination of the driver's state and performance. The measures of driver's state include percent eye closure, mouth shape, and head position. The state is captured via cameras and/or sensors installed in the driver's car. The measures of driver performance include lane tracking and tracking of distance between vehicles [88].

4.4.3   AT for Crime Risk

The regular panic button is mainly functional in indoor environments (e.g., house, hospital, retirement facility) and is not extendable to outdoor. Advanced technology may help preventing certain crime situations, particularly abuse and violence in outdoor environment, through the use of wearable devices (e.g., smartphone and bracelet). Similar to the regular panic button, Assistive Technology for crime risk is based on sending a request from user through smartphone or bracelet when a person feels unsafe. This request that contains the user location can be delivered to an emergency contact (e.g., emergency center, family, and friends). It is also possible to record the audio and even open the camera video to register the situation. Other accessories can be integrated to smartphone such as an alarm or LED light to disorient the attacker. Whistl [91] is a special iPhone case connected to a mobile application on smartphone via Bluetooth. This special case is equipped with 120 dB alarm and 90 lumen strobing LED which can be immediately activated by the user to disorient the attacker in case of a dangerous situation. The application can alert friends and the police instantly. Safelet, created by Dutch company Everfind, is a simple safety bracelet that allows elderly people to send out an alert whenever they feel that they are in danger [72].

4.4.4   AT for Psychological Related Risks

Psychological related risks are due to several factors including stress, depression, loneliness, and sedentary life. Therefore, assistive technology for psychological related risks are based on detecting emotional status of elderly people and provide suitable interventions in order to prevent or minimize psychological related risks and mainly suicide risk. Stress detection enables to intervene in an early stage. The basic principles of stress detection in the literature are monitoring health parameters (e.g., skin conductance, respiration, heart rate, cardiac signals), then applying various artificial intelligence techniques to separate stress from other emotional status (e.g., relaxation) [64].

Only few assistive technologies have been developed to allow elderly people to keep in touch with their friends and family. These applications are not necessarily designed to prevent any specific disease process, but rather, to promote the healthy behaviors of users. A part of the applications in this category incorporate gaming technology to provide motivations for improving health [32]. Other systems are designed to motivate social interaction. The Teleassistance platform enables elderly people to keep in touch with friends and family members through videoconference service [20].

The gerontechnological systems that motivate elderly people to increase their physical or social activities, are considered within the category of well-being m-health applications. QueFaire is an adaptable context-aware activity promoting system to improve well-being by recommending the most likeable activities for an elderly person according to his/her profile/preferences [69]. MELCO is an ICT system that targets elderly people and tries to increase their social activities and monitor their health at the same time. The system enables to build a virtual social network among people, their families, and friends. Through a mobile phone application people are offered several pre-recorded social activities in an outdoor environment [59].

5   Conclusion and Future Directions

Nowadays, there is great pressure to handle the situation of elderly people in our society, since most of them live alone and with no accompanying family member. Therefore, a solution as moving to healthcare facility can take place to support and provide care to them, however some negative emotional and economic impacts may arrive and this solution may not be the best. Thus, assistive technology is an advantageous option for elderly people. This population sector is vulnerable to several major risks. We presented in this paper the results of our study on risks affecting elderly people in outdoor activities of daily living. The results of our study reveal that the most addressed risks by ICT are fall, wandering, and health issues. We reviewed in this paper these three major risks, and discussed related assistive technology. We also proposed a framework that illustrates the logic of handling risks using assistive technology. In this paper, we also reviewed other risks affecting elderly people in outdoor environment and briefly discussed their related assistive technology (traffic accidents, fatigue, mistreatment, abuse, crime, and psychological related risks).

The recent advances in pervasive, mobile and wearable technologies opened new perspectives to enhance elderly people quality of life, by assisting them in activities of daily living. We have presented in this paper interesting representative examples of recent assistive technology linked to outdoor risks. Still, these solutions are fragmented and more research on combined ubiquitous assistance services is needed to cover the need spectrum of elderly people. An interesting proposition could be an integrated service platform that accommodates safety assurance, health support services, and daily activity assistance. Such platform could take care of anomalous events detection, daily activities tracking/assistance, and health status monitoring. This platform could leverage stationary sensors deployed in living environments and mobile sensing artifacts carried by elderly people. In this context, our team aims to provide elderly people with a comprehensive assistive system that manages risks. We are working on extending our mobile platform named PhonAge [4] to manage outdoor risk situations.

References

1. Abbate, S., Avvenuti, M., Bonatesta, F., Cola, G., Corsini, P., Vecchio, A.: A smartphone-based fall detection system. Pervasive Mob. Comput. **8**(6), 883–899 (2012)
2. Abdulrazak, B., Roy, P., Gouin-Vallerand, C., Belala, Y., Giroux, S.: Micro context-awareness for autonomic pervasive computing. Int. J. Bus. Data Commun. Networking (IJBDCN) **7**(2), 49–69 (2011)
3. Abdulrazak, B., Giroux, S., Mokhtari, M., Bouchard, B., Pigot, H.: Towards Useful Services for Elderly and People with Disabilities. Lecture Notes in Computer Science, vol. 6719. Springer, Heidelberg (2011)
4. Abdulrazak, B., Malik, Y., Arab, F., Reid, S.: PhonAge: adapted smartphone for aging population. In: Biswas, J., Kobayashi, H., Wong, L., Abdulrazak, B., Mokhtari, M. (eds.) ICOST 2013. LNCS, vol. 7910, pp. 27–35. Springer, Heidelberg (2013)
5. Abou-Raya, S., ElMeguid, L.A.: Road traffic accidents and the elderly. Geriatr. Gerontol. Int. **9**(3), 290–297 (2009)
6. Acampora, G., Cook, D.J., Rashidi, P., Vasilakos, A.V.: A survey on ambient intelligence in healthcare. Proc. IEEE **101**(12), 2470–2494 (2013)
7. Avlund, K.: Fatigue in older adults: an early indicator of the aging process? Aging Clin. Exp. Res. **22**(2), 100–115 (2010)
8. Bächlin, M., Plotnik, M., Roggen, D., Maidan, I., Hausdorff, J.M., Giladi, N., Troster, G.: Wearable assistant for Parkinson's disease patients with the freezing of gait symptom. IEEE Trans. Inf Technol. Biomed. **14**(2), 436–446 (2010)
9. Barnsley, L., McCluskey, A., Middleton, S.: What people say about travelling outdoors after their stroke: a qualitative study. Aust. Occup. Ther. J. **59**(1), 71–78 (2012)
10. Baum, A., Polsusnzy, D.: Health psychology: mapping biobehavioral contributions to health and illness. Annu. Rev. Psychol. **50**, 137–163 (1999)

11. Beard, J.R.: Neighborhood characteristics and disability in older adults. J. Gerontol. B Psychol. Sci. Soc. Sci. **64**(2), 252–257 (2009)
12. Beauvais, B.S., Rialle, V. Sablier, J.: MyVigi: An Android Application to Detect Fall and Wandering (2012)
13. Billette, J., Janz, T.: Living arrangements of seniors. Canadian Census (2011)
14. Blazer, G.: Depression in late life: review and commentary. J. Gerontol. A **58**(3), 249–265 (2003)
15. Brubaker, T.H.: Family Relationships in Later Life, vol. 64. Sage Publications, Newbury Park (1990)
16. Bruce, L., Pearson, L.: Designing an intervention to prevent suicide: PROSPECT (prevention of suicide in primary care elderly: collaborative trial). Dialogues Clin. Neurosci. **1**(2), 100–112 (1999)
17. Cao, Y., Yang, Y., Liu, W.: E-FallD: a fall detection system using android-based smartphone. In: The 9th IEEE International Conference on Fuzzy Systems and Knowledge Discovery (FSKD), pp. 1509–1513 (2012)
18. Chiarini, G., Ray, P., Akter, S., Masella, C., Ganz, A.: mHealth technologies for chronic diseases and elders: a systematic review. IEEE J. Sel. Areas Commun. **31**(9), 6–18 (2013)
19. Clarke, W.: Top 10 Vehicles for Seniors for (2014). http://www.edmunds.com/car-reviews/top-10/top-10-vehicles-for-seniors-for-2014.html
20. Cruz-Martín, E., del Árbol Pérez, L.P., Fernández González, L.C.: The teleassistance platform: an innovative technological solution in face of the ageing population problem. In: The 6th International Conference of the International Society for Gerontechnology
21. Dai, J., Bai, X., Yang, Z., Shen, Z., Xuan, D.: PerFallD: a pervasive fall detection system using mobile phones. In: The 8th IEEE International Conference on Pervasive Computing and Communications Workshops (PERCOM Workshops), pp. 292–297 (2010)
22. Butler-Jones, D.: Report on Seniors' Falls in Canada. Division of Aging and Seniors, Public Health Agency of Canada, Ottawa (2005)
23. Degen, T., Jaeckel, H., Rufer, M., Wyss, S.: SPEEDY: a fall detector in a wrist watch. In: ISWC, pp. 184–189 (2003)
24. De Jager, D., Wood, A. L., Merrett, G. V., Al-Hashimi, B. M., O'Hara, K., Shadbolt, N. R., Hall, W.: A low-power, distributed, pervasive healthcare system for supporting memory. In: Proceedings of the First ACM MobiHoc Workshop on Pervasive Wireless Healthcare (2011)
25. DiCarlo, L.A.: Role for direct electronic verification of pharmaceutical ingestion in pharmaceutical development. Contemp. Clin. Trials **33**, 593–600 (2012)
26. Douglas, A., Letts, L., Richardson, J.: A systematic review of accidental injury from fire, wandering and medication self-administration errors for older adults with and without dementia. Arch. Gerontol. Geriatr. **52**(1), 1–10 (2011)
27. Doukas, C., Metsis, V., Becker, E., Le, Z., Makedon, F., Maglogiannis, I.: Digital cities of the future: extending@ home assistive technologies for the elderly and the disabled. Telematics Inform. **28**(3), 176–190 (2011)
28. Ekmann, A., Petersen, I., Mänty, M., Christensen, K., Avlund, K.: Fatigue, general health, and ischemic heart disease in older adults. J. Gerontol. A Biol. Sci. Med. Sci. **68**(3), 279–285 (2013)
29. El-Bendary, N., Tan, Q., Pivot, F.C., Lam, A.: Fall detection and prevention for the elderly: a review of trends and challenges. Int. J. Smart Sens. Intell. Syst. **6**(3), 1230–1266 (2013)
30. Ferreira, F., Dias, F., Braz, J., Santos, R., Nascimento, R., Ferreira, C., Martinho, R.: Protege: a mobile health application for the elder-caregiver monitoring paradigm. Procedia Technol. **9**, 1361–1371 (2013)

31. Finkel, S.I., Silva, J.C.E., Cohen, G., Miller, S., Sartorius, N.: Behavioral and psychological signs and symptoms of dementia: a consensus statement on current knowledge and implications for research and treatment. Int. Psychogeriatr. **8**(S3), 497–500 (1997)

32. Gerling, K., Livingston, I., Nacke, L., Mandryk, R.: Full-body motion-based game interaction for older adults. In: Proceedings of the ACM SIGCHI Conference on Human Factors in Computing Systems, pp. 1873–1882 (2012)

33. Goergen, T., Beaulieu, M.: Critical concepts in elder abuse research. Int. Psychogeriatr. **25** (8), 1217–1228 (2013)

34. Guo, X., Duan, X., Gao, H., Huang, A., Jiao, B.: An ECG monitoring and alarming system based on android smart phone. Commun. Network **5**(03), 584–589 (2013)

35. Helal, A., Mokhtari, M., Abdulrazak, B.: The engineering handbook of smart technology for aging, disability, and independence. Wiley, New Jersey (2008)

36. Hellström, Y., Persson, G., Hallberg, I.R.: Quality of life and symptoms among older people living at home. J. Adv. Nurs. **48**(6), 584–593 (2004)

37. Jacobsen, A., Kent, M., Lee, M., Mather, M.: America's aging population. Popul. Bull. **66** (1), 1–20 (2011)

38. Kelsey, J.L., Berry, S.D., Procter-Gray, E., Quach, L., Nguyen, U.S.D., Li, W., Kiel, D.P., Lipsitz, L.A., Hannan, M.T.: Indoor and outdoor falls in older adults are different: the maintenance of balance, independent living, intellect, and zest in the elderly of boston study. J. Am. Geriatr. Soc. **58**(11), 2135–2141 (2010)

39. Khaddaj-Mallat, H., Yared, R., Abdulrazak, B.: Assistive technology for risks affecting elderly people in outdoor environment. In: (ICT4AgeingWell'2015) (2015)

40. Klasnja, P., Pratt, W.: Healthcare in the pocket: mapping the space of mobile-phone health interventions. J. Biomed. Inform. **45**(1), 184–198 (2012)

41. Klaus, P.A.: Crimes against persons age 65 or older, 1993–2002, US Department of Justice, Office of Justice Programs, Bureau of Justice Statistics (2005)

42. Krueger, K.R., Wilson, R.S., Kamenetsky, J.M., Barnes, L.L., Bienias, J.L., Bennett, D.A.: Social engagement and cognitive function in old age. Exp. Aging Res. **35**(1), 45–60 (2009)

43. Li, J., Zhou, H., Zuo, D., Hou, K.M., De Vaulx, C.: Ubiquitous health monitoring and real-time cardiac arrhythmias detection: a case study. Bio-Med. Mater. Eng. **24**(1), 1027–1033 (2014)

44. Li, Q., Stankovic, J.A., Hanson, M.A., Barth, A.T., Lach, J., Zhou, G.: Accurate, fast fall detection using gyroscopes and accelerometer-derived posture information. In: The 6th International Workshop on Wearable and Implantable Body Sensor Networks, pp. 138–143 (2009)

45. Lin, C.C., Chiu, M.J., Hsiao, C.C., Lee, R.G., Tsai, Y.S.: Wireless health care service system for elderly with dementia. IEEE Trans.Inf. Technol. Biomed. **10**(4), 696–704 (2006)

46. Lin, Q., Zhang, D., Chen, L., Ni, H., Zhou, X.: Managing elders' wandering behavior using sensors-based solutions: a survey. Int. J. Gerontol. **8**(2), 49–55 (2014)

47. Lithwick, M., Beaulieu, M., Gravel, S., Straka, M.: The mistreatment of older adults: perpetrator-victim relationships and interventions. J. Elder Abuse Negl. **11**(4), 95–112 (2000)

48. Loraine, A., Cole, S., Goodkind, D., He, W.: 65 + in the United States. U.S. Census Bureau, Government Printing Office, Washington, DC (2014)

49. Ludwig, W., Wolf, K.H., Duwenkamp, C., Gusew, N., Hellrung, N., Marschollek, M., Wagner, M., Haux, R.: Health-enabling technologies for the elderly–an overview of services based on a literature review. Comput. Methods Programs Biomed. **106**(2), 70–78 (2012)

50. Lv, Z., Xia, F., Wu, G., Yao, L., Chen, Z.: iCare: a mobile health monitoring system for the elderly. In: Proceedings of the IEEE/ACM International Conference on Green Computing

and Communications and International Conference on Cyber, Physical and Social Computing, pp. 699–705 (2010)

51. Mänty, M., de Leon, C.F.M., Rantanen, T., Era, P., Pedersen, A.N., Ekmann, A., Avlund, K.: Mobility-related fatigue, walking speed, and muscle strength in older people. J. Gerontol. A Biol. Sci. Med. Sci. **67**(5), 523–529 (2012)
52. Martel, L., Menard, F.: Statistics Canada. Canadian Census, Demography Division (2011)
53. McGillicuddy, J., Weiland, A., Frenzel, R., Mueller, M., Brunner-Jackson, B., Taber, D.: Patient attitudes toward mobile phone-based health monitoring: questionnaire study among kidney transplant recipients. J. Med. Internet Res. **15**(1), e6 (2013)
54. Morrow-Howell, N., Putnam, M., Lee, Y.S., Greenfield, J.C., Inoue, M., Chen, H.: An investigation of activity profiles of older adults. J. Gerontol. B Psychol. Sci. Soc. Sci. **69**(5), 809–821 (2014)
55. Mougiakakou, S. G., Kouris, I., Iliopoulou, D., Vazeou, A., Koutsouris, D.: Mobile technology to empower people with diabetes mellitus: design and development of a mobile application. In: The 9th International Conference on Information Technology and Applications in Biomedicine, ITAB, pp. 1–4 (2009)
56. Mubashir, M., Shao, L., Seed, L.: A survey on fall detection: principles and approaches. Neurocomputing **100**, 144–152 (2013)
57. National Institute of Aging: Workshop on Unexplained Fatigue in the Elderly. Workshop Summary. National Institute of Aging (2007)
58. Nehmer, J., Becker, M., Karshmer, A., Lamm, R.: Living assistance systems: an ambient intelligence approach. In: Proceedings of the 28th International Conference on Software Engineering, pp. 43–50 (2006)
59. Neocleous, G.: Ageing and information communication technology: the case of melco in cyprus. Neocleous **9**(32), 13–32 (2013)
60. Ogorevc, A., Lončarevič, B.: iHELP emergency care network. In: 37th International Convention Information and Communication Technology, Electronics and Microelectronics (MIPRO) (2014)
61. Olla, P., Shimskey, C.: mHealth taxonomy: a literature survey of mobile health applications. Health Technol. **4**(4), 299–308 (2015)
62. Ozcan, K., Member, S., Mahabalagiri, A.K.: Automatic fall detection and activity classification by a wearable embedded smart camera. Dept. Electr. Eng. Comput. Sci. **3** (2), 125–136 (2013)
63. Parnes, R.B.: GPS Technology and Alzheimer's Disease: Novel Use for an Existing Technology (2003)
64. Pauws, S.C., Biehl, M.: Insightful stress detection from physiology modalities using learning vector quantization. Neurocomputing **151**, 873–882 (2015)
65. Pedone, C., Chiurco, D., Scarlata, S., Incalzi, R.A.: Efficacy of multiparametric telemonitoring on respiratory outcomes in elderly people with COPD: a randomized controlled trial. BMC Health Serv. Res. **13**(1), 82 (2013)
66. Penninx, B., Milaneschi, Y., Lamers, F., Vogelzangs, N.: Understanding the somatic consequences of depression: biological mechanisms and the role of depression symptom profile. BMC Med. **11**(1), 129 (2013)
67. Perälä, S., Mäkelä, K., Salmenaho, A., Latvala, R.: Technology for elderly with memory impairment and wandering risk. E-Health Telecommun. Syst. Netw. **2**(1), 13–22 (2013)
68. Pioggia, G., Tartarisco, G., Ricci, G., Volpi, L., Siciliano, G., De Rossi, D., Bonfiglio, S.: A wearable pervasive platform for the intelligent monitoring of muscular fatigue. In: The 10th IEEE International Conference on Intelligent Systems Design and Applications (ISDA), pp. 132–135 (2010)

69. Ponce, V., Deschamps, J.-P., Giroux, L.-P., Salehi, F., Abdulrazak, B.: QueFaire: context-aware in-person social activity recommendation system for active aging. In: Geissbühler, A., Demongeot, J., Mokhtari, M., Abdulrazak, B., Aloulou, H. (eds.) ICOST 2015. LNCS, vol. 9102, pp. 64–75. Springer, Heidelberg (2015)

70. Ramage-Morin, P.L.: Motor vehicle accident deaths, 1979 to 2004. Health Rep. **19**, 45–51 (2008)

71. Rashidi, P., Mihailidis, A.: A survey on ambient-assisted living tools for older adults. IEEE J. Biomed. Health Inf. **17**(3), 579–590 (2013)

72. Safelet. http://www.safelet.com/

73. Substance Abuse and Mental Health Services Administration and Administration on Aging (AoA): Behavioral health Technical Assistance Center (2012)

74. Schwickert, L., Becker, C., Lindemann, U., Maréchal, C., Bourke, A., Chiari, L., Helbostad, J.L., Zijlstra, W., Aminian, K., Todd, C., Bandinelli, S., Klenk, J.: Fall detection with body-worn sensors. Z. Gerontol. Geriatr. **46**(8), 706–719 (2013)

75. Shen, J., Barbera, J., Shapiro, M.: Distinguishing sleepiness and fatigue: focus on definition and measurement. Sleep Med. Rev. **10**(1), 63–76 (2006)

76. Simoni-Wastila, L., Yang, H.K.: Psychoactive drug abuse in older adults. Am. J. Geriatr. Pharmacother. **4**, 380–394 (2006)

77. Sperling, A., Aisen, S., Beckett, A., Bennett, A., Craft, S., Fagan, M., Phelps, H.: Toward defining the preclinical stages of alzheimer's disease: recommendations from the national institute on aging-alzheimer's association workgroups on diagnostic guidelines for alzheimer's disease. Alzheimer Dement. **7**(3), 280–292 (2011)

78. Sposaro, F., Tyson, G.: iFall: an android application for fall monitoring and response. Conf. Proc. Ann. Int. Conf. IEEE Eng. Med. Biol. Soc. **2009**, 6119–6122 (2009)

79. Sposaro, F., Danielson, J. Tyson, G.: iWander: an android application for dementia patients. In: Annual International Conference of the IEEE Engineering in Medicine and Biology Society (EMBC), pp. 3875–3878 (2010)

80. Stegemann, S., Baeyens, J.P., Cerreta, F., Chanie, E., Löfgren, A., Maio, M., Thesing-Bleck, E.: Adherence measurement systems and technology for medications in older patient populations. Eur. Geriatr. Med. **3**(4), 254–260 (2012)

81. Ströhle, A.: Physical activity, exercise, depression and anxiety disorders. J. Neural Transm. **116**(6), 777–784 (2009)

82. Sugiyama, T., Thompson, C.W.: Environmental support for outdoor activities and older people's quality of life. J. Hous. Elderly **19**, 167–185 (2006)

83. Taleb, T., Fadlullah, Z. M., Bottazzi, D., Nasser, N., Chen, Y.: A context-aware middleware-level solution towards a ubiquitous healthcare system. In: The IEEE International Conference on Wireless and Mobile Computing, Networking and Communications, WIMOB, pp. 61–66 (2009)

84. Tervonen, J., Asghar, Z., Parviainen, E., Nissinen, H., Ylipelto, M., Shikur, H., Pulli, P., Yamamoto, G.: Design for all case study: a navigation aid for elderly persons. In: IEEE Conference on Engineering, Technology and Innovation (ICE) (2014)

85. Ting, P.H., Hwang, J.R., Doong, J.L., Jeng, M.C.: Driver fatigue and highway driving: a simulator study. Physiol. Behav. **94**(3), 448–453 (2008)

86. Tong, L., Song, Q., Ge, Y., Liu, M.: HMM-based human fall detection and prediction method using tri-axial accelerometer. IEEE Sens. J. **13**(5), 1849–1856 (2013)

87. Toshio, O., Iwasaki, N.: Innovative applications and strategy on ICT applications for aging society: case study of Japan for silver ICT innovations. In: Proceedings of the 7th ACM International Conference on Theory and Practice of Electronic Governance (2013)

88. Wang, Q., Yang, J., Ren, M., Zheng, Y.: Driver fatigue detection: a survey. In: The Proceedings of the IEEE Intelligent Control and Automation, vol. 2, pp. 8587–8591 (2006)

89. Wennberg, H., Hydén, C., Ståhl, A.: Barrier-free outdoor environments: older peoples' perceptions before and after implementation of legislative directives. Transp. Policy **17**(6), 464–474 (2010)

90. Wick, J.Y., LaFleur, J.: Fatigue: implications for the elderly. Consultant Pharmacist **22**(7), 566–578 (2007)

91. Wood, C.: Whistl iPhone case aims to prevent and deter assaults (2014). http://www.gizmag.com/whistl-iphone-case-assault-prevention/34169/

92. World Health Organization (WHO), International classification of functioning, disability and health: (ICF) (2002)

93. World Health Organization (WHO), Preventing suicide: a global imperative (2014)

94. Xiao, B., Asghar, M. Z., Jamsa, T., Pulii, P.: "Canderoid": a mobile system to remotely monitor travelling status of the elderly with dementia. In: The International Joint Conference on Awareness Science and Technology and Ubi-Media Computing (iCAST-UMEDIA), pp. 648–654 (2013)

95. Yamada, Y., Denkinger, M.D., Onder, G., Finne-Soveri, H., van der Roest, H., Vlachova, M., Tomas, R., Jacob, G., Roberto, B., Topinkova, E.: Impact of dual sensory impairment on onset of behavioral symptoms in european nursing homes: results from the services and health for elderly in long-term care study. J. Am. Med. Directors Assoc. **16**(4), 329–333 (2014)

96. Yang, Y.C., McClintock, M.K., Kozloski, M., Li, T.: Social isolation and adult mortality: the role of chronic inflammation and sex differences. J. Health Soc. Behav. **54**(2), 183–203 (2013)

97. Yu, X.: Approaches and principles of fall detection for elderly and patient. In: The 10th International Conference on e-health Networking, Applications and Services. HealthCom, pp. 42–47 (2008)

98. Zhao, Z., Chen, Y., Wang, S., Chen, Z.: Fallalarm: smart phone based fall detecting and positioning system. Procedia Comput. Sci. **10**, 617–624 (2012)

Toward Context-Aware Smart Oven
to Prevent Cooking Risks in Kitchen
of Elderly People

Rami Yared[⊠] and Bessam Abdulrazak

Université de Sherbrooke, 2500, boul. de l'Université, Sherbrooke, QC, Canada
{rami.yared,bessam.abdulrazak}@usherbrooke.ca

Abstract. Active life style promotes healthy aging. Cooking, particularly, is an important activity of daily living for elderly people. However, cooking is accompanied with several risks for this population category due to the aging related decline. Assistive technology is a promising solution to assist elderly people and enhance their safety. We introduce in this paper a context-aware cooking-safe environment, an innovative assistive technology to enhance safety of elderly people while cooking. We mainly focus in this paper on the hardware architecture of our system. The context is gathered via sensors deployed in kitchen environment. The system is composed of sensor nodes, microcontroller, and a computing unit. We also introduce in this paper a solution for sensors positioning and system integration in a real-world cooking environment. Furthermore, we present the results of sensors testing in real-world configurations.

Keywords: Risk · Hazard · Safety · Cooking · Prevention · Fire · Burn · Intoxication · Gas · Smoke · Sensor · Activities of daily living · Elderly people

1 Introduction

Safety of elderly people while cooking remains a big concern, since aging is a process associated with cognitive decline and memory impairment. The kitchen is the second place where the majority of domestic accidents occur, and in particular the oven presents the main source of fire accidents in residences [3, 14]. Studies revealed that unattended cooking is the main leading factor responsible for fire in the kitchen [3, 12]. Following is an example that illustrates the gravity of the situation [1]. Elderly people often put a pot on an oven burner, and engage in other activities (e.g., watch television, sleep, call another person) forgetting the pot on burner. This situation, which is due to attention and memory problems, may cause fire accident and lead to catastrophic results (e.g., death of the elderly people). Hence, enabling kitchen safety is a major factor for elderly people independent living.

The need of providing safety for elderly people at home becomes more significant because of the increasing number of elderly people around the world, and particularly in the developed countries. In Canada, the proportion of elderly people aged 65 years or over will represent between 23 % and 25 % of the population by 2036, and between 24 % and 28 % by 2061 [5, 9, 13]. In Japan, the population of 65 year-old was about

© Springer International Publishing Switzerland 2015
M. Helfert et al. (Eds.): ICT4AgeingWell 2015, CCIS 578, pp. 57–77, 2015.
DOI: 10.1007/978-3-319-27695-3_4

25.1 % of the total population in 2013, and will be 40 % in 2050, which is the highest ratio of aging population in the world [17]. In the United States, the number of elderly people is also on the rise: in 2010, there were 40.3 million people aged 65 and above, comprising 13 % of the overall population. This proportion is 12 times higher than it was in 1900, when this group constituted only 4.1 % of the population. By 2050, projections indicate the population over 65 will comprise 20.9 % of the population in the United States [11]. In Europe, by 2025 more than 20 % of population will be 65 or over, with a particularly rapid increase in the number of over 80 s. In the United States, 40 % of women and 19 % of men aged 65 years and older, live alone and do not have anyone in the home to assist with activities of daily living, provide care when they are sick, or to assist with home maintenance [10].

Elderly people prefer stay independent at their home while aging. Due to the aging related decline, elderly people are strongly concerned by cooking associated risks (e.g., fire, burn or intoxication) [1]. Therefore, elderly people are often forced to stop cooking or completely move to a nursing home or a healthcare facility to prevent dangerous situations. Urgent intervention is required to provide a solution that prevents risks in daily life activities. A possible solution to enable elderly people stay at home is to be accompanied by a family member or a caregiver for cooking activity. However, this solution is not practical due to independency and privacy issues. In addition, it has several drawbacks such as high cost and a shortage of qualified professionals. It also requires that elderly people accept the idea of being not completely autonomous needing help. These factors negatively affect the moral situation of elderly people and consequently complicate the cognitive deficiencies recovery [16]. Therefore, assistive technology is a potential alternative to enhance safety at home.

We present in this paper our attempt to establish a preventive approach for enhancing safety of elderly people, with a cooking-safe system that proactively reacts to hazards in order to prevent cooking associated risks. We believe that providing elderly people with safe environments will enable them to stay home longer before being forced to move to a nursing facility, and consequently leads to better quality of life. We envision a context-aware cooking-safe system composed of sensor nodes that enable collecting context and situation around oven [1]. The context is processed to prevent risks, based on the results of our insightful experimental cooking risk analysis. We present the hardware architecture of our cooking-safe system, and discuss the selection of the sensors that has been inferred from our risk analysis and experiential studies. We present the results of our experimental study including testing sensors in real-world environment. Based on the gathered context, the system monitors and measures the pertinent parameters around oven. The pertinent parameters are extracted based on our extensive risk analysis and assessment experimental results [20].

The remainder of the paper is organized as follows. Section 2 presents the related work. Section 3 presents a brief summary of our cooking-risk analysis during cooking, and the hardware architecture of our cooking-safe system. Section 3 discusses the selected sensors that enable collecting context and that constitute the basic building block of the system, sensors positioning in the cooking environment, and the results of the sensors testing. Finally, Sect. 4 concludes the paper and discusses future work.

2   Related Work

"Risk" and "Hazard" are generally used interchangeably in the literature. We distinguish between risk and hazard [1, 20]. We define Risk as the potential of occurrence of an event that yields unwanted results, and Hazard as a contextual reason that causes a Risk. Cooking activity is accompanied with several potential hazardous contexts. Almost everybody who cooks has forgotten a dish (e.g., pizza) in the oven to burn, which led to a smoke and activation of an alarm. This hazardous context may lead to fire, and this context is more critical in case of elderly people due to memory impairments. Statistics show that elderly people forget often a pot on burner, which may cause several risks. The three major risks during cooking are fire, burn, and intoxication [20]. The literature reveals that existing research often addresses only one particular risk in cooking (fire), and there is no global solution for kitchen safety. To the best of our knowledge, no research work provides solutions to prevent burn or intoxication risks during cooking activities.

A basic existing solution to handle fire risk at home is installing fire alarms. The main concern of fire alarms is to detect fire occurrence quickly, so fire rescue agents can intervene in time. However, existing fire alarms have several drawbacks, particularly for elderly people. These people usually forget replacing alarm batteries regularly. In addition, fire alarms generate false alarms (e.g., in the presence of a small quantity of smoke generated by regular cooking). This situation disturbs elderly people, which increases their tendency to uninstall fire alarms at their homes. Lushaka et al. establish an elaborated system that relies on existing smoke alarms to detect a potential fire risk, and consequently, reacts by switching off oven power supply [12]. The system considers only fire risk and depends on existing smoke alarms. Doman et al. establish a system for assisting elderly people in the kitchen through video and audio [7]. This system reminds user to follow the correct steps when performing a cooking task, so it can possibly avoid cooking hazards, but it does not react when a dangerous situation occurs. Other intelligent assistive technologies are designed for people with cognitive deficiencies. Yahui et al. propose a design for a smart kitchen environment to assist elderly people suffering from dementia in cooking process. Using the system, caregivers remotely instruct users according to a cooking workflow. In addition, a visual surveillance system with multiple cameras enables to observe cooking conditions, and track user activities and object movement [19]. This system is not completely automatic, since it requires observer intervention and it is based on visual monitoring by cameras, which may be considered intrusive. Sanchez et al. establish a system that assists people in the kitchen and reacts when a potentially dangerous situation is detected [15]. The system detects rapid variations in temperature and smoke in the kitchen, and sends a notification (with camera shots) to the fire department and caregivers. In addition, the system activates exhaust fans and a fire extinguishing suppression system. A number of studies mention oven monitoring as a part of larger systems to track activities of daily living. Alwan et al. [4] measure oven usage and Wai et al. [18] propose detecting unsafe usage of the oven. Both systems use embedded temperature sensors to measure the burner status, ultrasonic sensors to detect the presence of a pot and electric current sensors to detect the oven usage and the levels of abnormality in the kitchen. Chen et al. propose a system that detects food ingredients based on visible-light cameras during cooking activities to ensure the healthy eating habits [6]. The three discussed systems either require modifications to the oven to install sensors, or use visible-light cameras. Visible-light cameras usually considered intrusive and are sensitive to cooking smoke. Yuan et al. develop an automated top oven monitoring system based on thermal camera to detect dangerous situations [21]. The system alerts user or caregiver when a dangerous situation occurs. The system does not require modifications to oven, so it fits any existing oven and respects user privacy, because it is based on thermal imaging instead of visible-light camera. Since the thermal camera does not process regular images, user privacy is preserved. However, the thermal camera has significant limitations since it is sensitive to cooking heat and smoke.

Few electrical cooking devices equipped with limited safety features are available in the market. For example, Electrolux INSPIRO oven contains programmable cooking modes. According to the selected cooking mode, the oven calculates cooking time and temperature. TMIO society commercializes ovens with tactile screen, and network connection to be remotely controlled. Numerous manufactures integrate LEDs to indicate that an oven surface is hot to prevent burn. However, the concentration of elderly people is mainly on the cooking task itself and she/he may not notice the lightening LED. Generally speaking, safety measures are partially considered in the existing commercial cooking devices. StoveGuard, SafeCook and HomeSensor propose a timer system to switch off an oven if there is no attendance after certain programmed time. Still, risks may occur within this period of time.

To summarize, existing systems propose numerous interesting features to manage risks at home. However, they have several limitations. They focus on aid for only one specific risk situation, they need to be programmed for each type of use and each time they are used (thereby providing elevated risks for variety of use or frequency of use), and also they provide elevated risks in the case of cognitive deficiencies. Therefore, performing a new extensive risk analysis on cooking safety is needed to build a robust cooking-safe system.

3   Research and Methodology

The aim of our team is to build a cooking-safe system that provides a preventive approach for enhancing safety in the kitchen. In order to build our system, we adopted three phases:

- Phase 1: we started by performing risk analysis and assessments during cooking. We performed our risk analysis and assessment in two phases. First, we reviewed literature to study the characteristics of the existing solutions for safety and risk analysis during cooking. We also extracted the pertinent parameters of cooking risks.
- Phase 2: based on our results of the risk analysis and assessment (Phase 1), we determined the pertinent parameters to monitor during cooking. Then, we select the appropriate sensors for the cooking-safe system based on the results of the risk analysis and assessment. We integrated these sensors and build a prototype of the

cooking-safe system. After that, we investigated several possible sensor positioning solutions, in order to select the most appropriate in a real-world cooking environment.

- Phase 3: we tested the sensors to determine the capacities and limitations of the selected sensors in real-world environment.

Following, we present in details each phase of our study.

3.1   Phase 1: Risk Analysis and Assessment During Cooking

The goal of this phase is to establish the relation between the contextual parameters and triggering risks. In order to focus only on sources of risks, independently from oven characteristics (e.g., gas factors related to gas oven), we used an electrical oven. We investigated several hazardous contexts during cooking in order to extract, monitor, and measure the pertinent parameters related to cooking risks. We performed series of experiments that reflect the real-world cooking scenarios with varieties of cooking materials. Following are a summary of the studied parameters:

- **Fire:** we observed the Volatile Organic Compound (VOC) and Alcohol gases' concentration parameters in the cooking smoke.
- **Burn:** for both, burn risk by splash and by contacting hot objects, we observed the relative humidity, utensil temperature, burner temperature, and presence of object on burner.
- **Intoxication by gas/smoke:** we observed the concentration of CO gas parameter in the cooking smoke.

We present in the next sections a summary of our experimental results on risk analysis and assessment [20].

A. *Study on Fire Risk.* We observed cooking of the following food types: fish, meat, onion, peppers, and spaghetti. Also, we heated oil (50 ml of canola oil) in a frying pan for 8 min until oil starts to shudder. Following a summary of our experimental results on cooking risk analysis and assessment.

- There is a correlation between fire triggering and the concentrations of certain chemical components in the cooking smoke, so detection of fire would be possible.
- Using existing sensors allows fire risk detection.
- Performance of the tested sensors is more improved than the performance of existing fire detectors on the shelf.
- Our experimentations lead us to determine the pertinent contextual parameters to be monitored in order to detect fire triggering in early stage i.e., VOC (aldehydes, alcohols and acids), hydrocarbons, and inflammable gases.
- There are boundaries between normal and dangerous contextual situations during cooking, with respect to the concentrations of VOC and Alcohol gases in the cooking smoke, e.g., if alcohol concentration in the cooking smoke exceeds 200 ppm (parts per million) then, there is a potential fire risk situation.

B. Study on Burn Risk. We distinguish two types of burn during cooking: burn by splash of hot liquids, and burn by contacting hot objects. We performed 12 experiments to measure temperatures of cooking utensils when water boils: three with a kettle, three with a frying pan, and six with a saucepan. In addition, we investigated dangerous situations by heating empty frying pan and saucepan. Following are the results:

- *Results on Burn by contacting Hot Object*
  - It is possible to prevent burn by contacting hot object during cooking, by monitoring utensil temperature and burner temperature.
  - There are distinct thresholds between normal and dangerous contextual situations.
  - Based on our experimental study, we determined experimental threshold values to discriminate between normal and burn risk situations related to contacting with a hot burner or a hot utensil. The threshold values of burner and utensil temperatures to discriminate between normal and burn risk are 75°C and 45°C respectively.
  - It is required at first to detect the presence of a utensil on a burner, in order to start monitoring its temperature. If there is no object on burner, it is required to monitor burner temperature.
- *Results on Burn by Splash*
  - A slight increment in the Relative Humidity (%RH) before water simmers, means that there is a release of small quantity of steam, and indicates that there is an object heated on burner.
  - An increment of 5 %RH indicates that water is simmering, so the global water temperature is around 100°C. Therefore, rapid variations in the relative humidity is an important indicator of water temperature in a utensil, and consequently a potential splash burn risk.
  - Boiled water reaches a dangerous temperature after two minutes of boiling.
  - % RH increases 8 % for majority of food kinds.
  - An increment of 30 % RH indicates a potential high risk of splash burn.

C. Study on Intoxication by Gas/Smoke Risk. We used the same experiments presented in fire risk analysis, by cooking several types of food in normal and dangerous contextual situations (i.e., fish, sausage, heated oil).

- CO concentration is a parameter to be monitored around oven in order to prevent intoxication by gas/smoke during cooking. Our experimentations lead us to determine the pertinent parameter to be monitored in order to prevent intoxication by gas/smoke during cooking (i.e., CO gas concentration in the cooking smoke).
- There are boundaries between normal and intoxication risk situations during cooking. The concentration of CO in the cooking smoke was around 40 ppm in our experimentation. If CO concentration in the cooking smoke exceeds 800 ppm then, there is a potential intoxication risk. So, we determined the threshold value of CO concentrations in order to prevent intoxication by gas/smoke during cooking.

To conclude, we confirmed that the pertinent contextual parameters to be monitored and measured around oven as: Volatile Organic Compound (VOC), Alcohol, CO concentrations in the cooking smoke, relative humidity, utensil temperature, burner temperature, and the presence of a utensil on burner.

3.2 Phase 2: Hardware Architecture of the Cooking-Safe System and Sensor Selection

We propose a context-aware pervasive computing approach [2] to build a robust sensor-based system that addresses cooking safety. The system allows sensing contextual cooking activities and offering appropriate context-aware interventions. Determining a risk situation and the corresponding interventions are adaptable to user contextual needs.

The system is based on a smart environment infrastructure, especially sensors and actuators distributed in the kitchen area:

- Sensors are selected based on phase 1. They are installed around oven to perform context acquisition. They allow the system to infer the situation during cooking, or detect changes in the surrounding environment (e.g., smoke, burner temperature, utensil temperature, and presence of a utensil on burner).
- Actuators are distributed in the residence to ubiquitously alert user of a cooking risk situation. They provide feedback through screens, speakers, or flashing lights, and control appliances in the kitchen (such as switch off oven power). The actuators provide a wide range of possibilities for human-machine interaction including appropriate intervention for each detected risk situation, and an adapted reaction according to user needs.

The system proactively reacts to contextual hazards in order to prevent cooking associated risks. Figure 1 illustrates the hardware architecture of the cooking-safe system.

1. **Sensor Selection.** Each sensor is selected to monitor one of the identified contextual parameters (i.e., utensil temperature, burner temperature, utensil presence on burner, relative humidity, CO, Alcohol, VOC). The selected sensors are illustrated in Table 1. Our selection is also based on real-world integration requirements, which can be summarized as follows:

   - Integration requirements: In order to integrate sensor nodes in the cooking environment, sensors must be non-intrusive. The selected sensor technologies (i.e., based on electrochemical, metal-oxide-semi-conductor, infrared, ultrasonic, and resistive hygrometer) do not require contact to operate, and can be installed around the cooking activity without interfering with user movement.
   - Practicability requirements: Analogue output signals of the selected sensors are easy to acquire. For resistive and metal-oxide-semi-conductor sensors, resistance variations are translated to voltage. For electrochemical sensors electric current is transformed into voltage, which can be easily interfaced with microcontrollers. In addition, price and appropriate response time are other factors that motivate our selection of sensors.

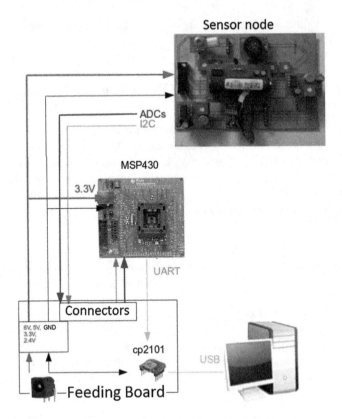

Fig. 1. Hardware architecture of the cooking-safe system.

2. ***Sensor Electrical Feeding***. The selected sensors require different electric feeding voltages, so a "feeding board" is designed to meet this requirement (Fig. 1). Electrical power is taken from the sector through a transformer, which delivers 12 V/1A as output. The four required electrical voltages (2.4 V, 3.3 V, 5 V, and 6 V) are obtained due to power regulators.

3. ***Microcontroller***. The selected microcontroller is MSP430 by Texas Instruments, because it has the following features: Analog to Digital Conversion (ADC), multiple input/output, and two communication ports (UART, I2C or SPI).

   The contextual sensory data is transmitted through cables ADC (5) and I2C (1), from sensor nodes to MSP430 microcontroller via the feeding board and then from the MSP430 microcontroller to the computing unit by one serial frame. The frame is routed to the computing unit via the cp2101 module, which converts serial frame to USB frame. The composition of the frame is illustrated in Fig. 2. Since environment variations are slow, we fixed the sampling period to one second. The frame is composed of the following attributes: ambient temperature, burner temperature, utensil temperature, relative humidity, distance between presence detection sensor and utensil (used to determine whether utensil is on burner or not), CO concentration, VOC concentration, and Alcohol concentration.

Table 1. The characteristics of the selected sensors.

Sensor	Contextual parameter	Technology	Unit	Response Time	Figure
Melexis MLX 90614	Ambient temperature and object temperature	Thermopile and infrared	°C	100ms	
SRF02	Object presence	Ultrasonic	cm	72ms	
Honeywell HIH-5030	Humidity	Resistive	--	5s	
Figaro TGS 5042	CO Carbone Monoxide	Electro-chemical	ppm	60s	
Figaro TGS 2620	Alcohol	Metal-Oxide semi-conductor	mV	20s	
MICS 5521	Volatile Organic Compounds (VOC)	Metal-Oxide semi-conductor	mV	10s	

4. ***Sensors Positioning***. The sensitivity of a sensor (output voltage) varies according to its position. Therefore, an appropriate positioning around the oven is required, to acquire precise sensor measurements and to satisfy the integration constraints presented above. We investigated several configurations and the following is our solution (Fig. 3). We placed on the oven hood level, the following sensors: humidity, VOC, Alcohol, CO, and temperature sensors. The temperature sensor on the hood is only to measure burner temperature (Fig. 4).

We placed on the workspace (20 cm to the left side of burner as illustrated in Fig. 4), the following sensors: distance measurement sensor for detecting the presence of utensil on burner and the temperature sensor to measure utensil temperature. This positioning configuration is non-intrusive as possible, in order not to disturb user movement and cooking habits. In addition, positioning sensors at the level of oven hood allows adequately monitoring the required parameters. In addition, the distance between oven hood and burner is adequate for acquiring

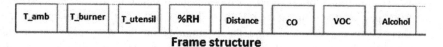

Frame structure

Fig. 2. Frame composed of sensory data from MSP430 to computing unit via serial port.

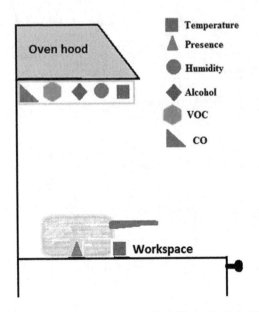

Fig. 3. Sensors positioning: Temperature (burner), Humidity, Alcohol, VOC, and CO on the oven hood level. Presence detection, and temperature (utensil) on the workspace.

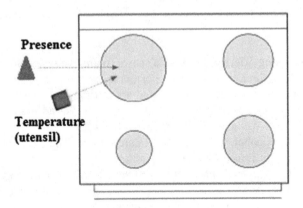

Fig. 4. Sensors positioning on the workspace (20 cm to the left side of burner): Distance measurement sensor for detecting the presence of a utensil on the burner and temperature sensor for measuring utensil temperature.

precise measurements from sensors based on the results of test for each sensor (Phase 3). The motivation behind positioning the distance measurement sensor on the workspace and not on the oven hood is that the distance (20 cm) is appropriate for this sensor measurements and the positioning on the workspace can avoid cooking heat. We also placed the temperature sensor (for measurement of utensil temperature) on the workspace, because of the low infrared emissivity of utensil's metal, which obstructs the measurements of this infrared sensor.

5. *System Building*. The cooking-safe system experimental kit has been built based on the following properties and features:

- Flexibility: possibility of adding new sensors if required. The sensor node is designed such that adding/removing sensors is easily performed.
- Simple physical installation: The sensors are integrated on a node such that the node can be placed in an alternative location if required. However, in this case, longer cables and appropriate sensor direction (for the presence detection sensor and the temperature sensor) are required.
- Non-intrusiveness: as the oven surface is free and the components of the system are placed in adequate positions as possible to monitor hazards and prevent risk situations. However, two sensors are placed in the workspace in addition to the microcontroller and a computing unit.

To summarize, we presented in this section of Phase 2, the selected sensors to collect context. We also discussed their characteristics, and the hardware architecture of our cooking-safe system. In addition, we discussed the positioning of the sensors in the environment, which satisfies the ergonomic and practical requirements. We discuss in the next phase (Phase 3), sensors testing and the limitations of the selected sensors in a real-world cooking environment.

3.3   Phase 3: System Testing

Sensor testing in real-world environment is crucial to validate the preventive approach and build a practical cooking-safe system. Therefore, a series of tests has been performed for each selected sensor. The objective is to investigate the behavior of each sensor in real-world, and thus determine its limitations. To illustrate the importance of the test let examine the following cases. Temperature, humidity, and gases change frequently around the oven. Furthermore, there is no single method of cooking in real-world. These factors may affect sensing data (e.g., putting a small utensil on a large burner, may affect the measurements of the presence detection sensor). Thus, various cooking behaviors have to be considered to obtain correct and precise measurements. Measurements of sensors are also affected by the position and orientation of sensors (e.g., the temperature sensor does not give the exact temperature if placed far from the monitored object).

Test Settings. The first test series was performed using one burner of the oven, using neither ventilation nor light above the oven because prior experiments revealed that sensory date are changing with oven ventilation and/or light. Utensils used are: saucepan, kettle (brilliant metal), frying pan (opaque metal) illustrated in Fig. 5, for this series of tests.

The saucepan is smaller than the burner in order to study non-ideal situations. These cooking tools are selected to study the infrared emissivity between different metals, and explain different behaviors of the infrared sensor. Similar to Phase 1

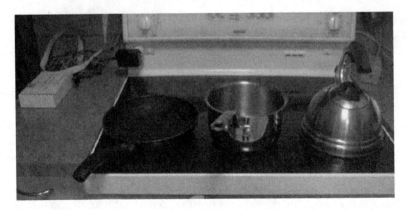

Fig. 5. Cooking utensils used for testing sensors.

concerning fire risk analysis, we performed in this phase experimentations of cooking several kinds of food: fish, meat, onion, peppers, and spaghetti, in addition to heating oil (50 ml of canola oil) in a frying pan for 8 min until oil starts to shudder. Following we present the results.

Test of VOC and Alcohol Sensors. We illustrate in Fig. 6 the distinct boundaries between normal and risk situations according to output voltages of the selected VOC

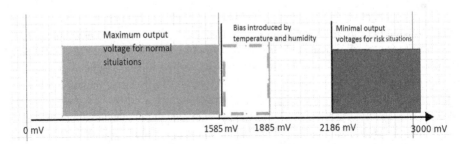

Fig. 6. Output voltages of Alcohol and VOC sensors in normal and dangerous situations.

and Alcohol sensors (Table 1), while cooking several kinds of food. The output voltages of VOC and Alcohol sensors in normal situations are as follows:

- In case of cooking hotdogs in a frying pan (Fig. 7), the maximal output voltages for normal situation are around 1500 mV ($\sim$ 150 ppm).
- In case of cooking fish, onion and peppers in a frying pan (Fig. 8), the maximal output voltages for normal situation are near 1000 mV ($\sim$ 100 ppm).
- In case of heating oil in a frying pan (e.g., for 8 min) (Fig. 9), the maximal output voltages for normal situation are near 2000 mV ($\sim$ 200 ppm) because heated oil releases more VOC and Alcohol in the cooking smoke compared to cooking meat, which releases more VOC and Alcohol than cooking fish and vegetables.

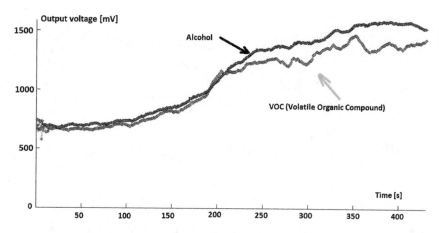

Fig. 7. Output voltages of VOC and Alcohol sensors when cooking hotdogs in a frying pan.

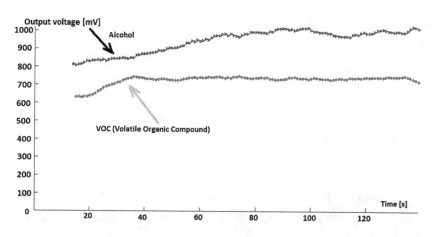

Fig. 8. Output voltages of VOC and Alcohol sensors when cooking fish in a frying pan.

Therefore, output voltages of VOC ($\sim$ ppm) and Alcohol sensors ($\sim$ ppm) allow determining fire risk. If output voltages are greater than 2000 mV (~ 200 ppm), then there is a potential fire risk.

Test of Presence Detection Sensor. The presence detection sensor is an ultrasonic sensor (Table 1) used to detect the context of utensil's presence on burner, based on measuring the distance between the sensor and the utensil. Sonar wave propagation depends on the propagation medium, so air variable conditions affect wave propagation. Ultrasonic sensor must compensate these effects in a variable environment. However, this sensor does not integrate such compensations. So, it has to be placed where the air is the most stable as possible; otherwise measurements will not be precise. We excluded certain places such as the oven hood (hot air, cooking gases, and evaporated water) and the control panel because the temperature will be very high.

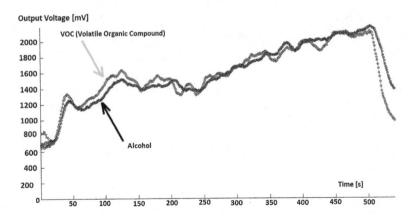

Fig. 9. Output voltages of VOC and Alcohol sensors when frying oil during 8 min.

Therefore, we positioned the presence detection sensor on the workspace around 20 cm to the left of the burner as illustrated in Fig. 10. We also found that the appropriate vertical positioning of the presence detection sensor is around 2 cm above workspace (Fig. 10). This vertical location allows detecting the presence of utensils with little height, like frying pan. If the sensor is vertically located lower than 2 cm then parasite may affect its measurements.

We tested the presence detection sensor by changing oven state (off/on), utensil type, utensil volume, and position of utensil on burner. The goal of changing the position of utensil on burner is to study the effect of heat on distance measurement.

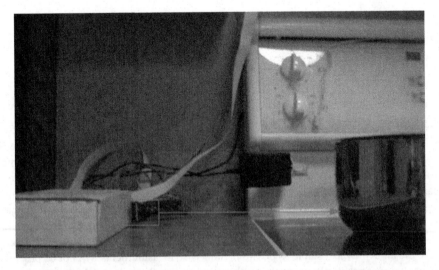

Fig. 10. The position of the presence detection sensor on the workspace.

Figure 11 shows seven different positions of the center of utensil. A series of measurements was performed, and yielded the following results:

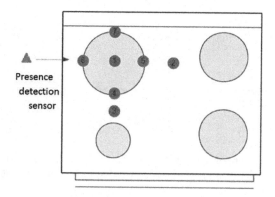

Fig. 11. Different positions of utensils on the burner.

- The very low position of the sensor is appropriate because this does not cause reflections. However, it must be horizontally oriented.
- To maintain the stable state of the sensor, a carton box covered it. Without these precautions, parasitic reflections appear.
- The measured values would be aberrant, if a utensil was placed further than 30 cm from the sensor.
- The experimental results show that the form and volume of a cooking utensil has no impact on distance measurement using the ultrasonic sensor.
- The obtained results show that ultrasonic wave propagation varies with surrounding air temperature. Each time there is hot air between sensor and object, the measurements becomes less reliable. This is the case when a utensil is not placed in the center of burner, or the case when a utensil is smaller than the burner.
- The distance measurements while cooking meat in a frying pan, which is larger than the burner and placed in the center of the burner are presented in Fig. 12. The flow of hot air between the sensor and the pan is minimal and hence measurements of distance are reliable.
- Figure 13 presents variable distance measurements while heating water in a saucepan, which is smaller than the burner and placed in the center of the burner.

The reason for unreliable measurements is that the exterior of the burner heats the surrounding air between the sensor and the utensil. Table 2 presents different distance measurements between the presence detection sensor and the center of different utensils placed in the seven positions illustrated in Fig. 11. The burner was (turned off/turned on to the maximum). The previous results reveal that it is possible to detect that an object is on burner. Variations in distance measurements according to the position of utensil allow us to determine a confidence zone, such that, if an object is placed in the interior of this zone, it is considered to be "on burner." The confidence zone is the outer rectangle (dark colored) illustrated in Fig. 14.

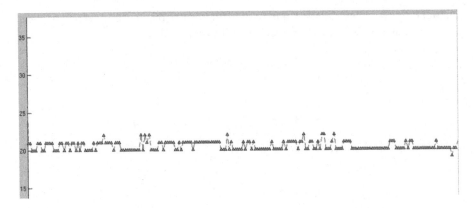

Fig. 12. Reliable distance measurements (cm) by the presence detection sensor while cooking meat in a frying pan larger than the burner and placed in the center of the burner.

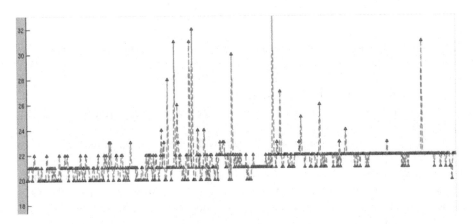

Fig. 13. Unreliable distance measurements (cm) by the presence detection sensor while heating water in a saucepan smaller than the burner and placed in the center of the burner.

Test of Temperature Sensor. Hot objects during cooking are utensils and burner. We performed 12 experiments to measure the temperature of utensils when water boils: three with a kettle, three with a frying pan, and six with a saucepan. In addition, we investigated dangerous situations by heating empty frying pan and saucepan. These experiments cover the majority of daily cooking situations. The motivation behind experimenting with boiled water is to overcome the measurements imprecision of the infrared sensor used to measure the temperature of a utensil since water boils at a known temperature (100°C). The results are presented in Table 3.

The imprecisions in measurement of utensil temperature are due to the low infrared emissivity of metals and to the heat of cooking that disturb the measurements of the infrared sensor.

Table 2. Distance measurements by the ultrasonic sensor according to utensil, its position on burner, and burner temperature.

Burner intensity	Situation	Kettle	Saucepan	Frying pan
		Distance measurements (cm)		
Turned off	1	26	25	23
	2	45	43	44
	3	90	70–90	95
	4	28	25	26
	5	34	34	35
	6	19	22	21
	7	27	25	21
Max	1	25	26	24–29
	2	47–64	49–72	42–125
	3	63–107	97–136	87–99
	4	24	27	26
	5	31–93	32–48	34–57
	6	21	19	18
	7	25	26	18

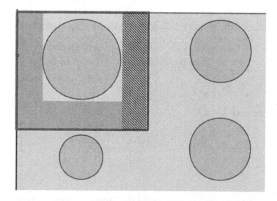

Fig. 14. The inner rectangle (light colored) zone represents the real "on-burner" zone. A utensil inside this zone is detected by the presence detection sensor. The outer rectangle (dark colored) zone represents the false positive zone of the sensor where a utensil is detected as "on-burner" and in reality it is outside burner. The shaded zone represents the dead zone of the sensor (Color figure online).

Test of Humidity Sensor. We performed a series of experiments focusing on context of heating liquid using different kinds of utensils: kettle and saucepan with/without lid for better understanding of the variations of the relative humidity (%RH) while liquid is boiling. In the first experiments, we measured the relative humidity using the hygrometer humidity sensor HIH-5030 by heating a utensil half-filled of water. As expected, the results illustrate that the variations of humidity depend on the quantity of the released steam. While the saucepan covered with lid, steam cannot be released.

Table 3. Experimental results of the measured utensil temperature when water boils.

Utensil	Experiment configuration	°C
Kettle	Center of burner	40
Frying pan	Center of burner	65
Saucepan	Bottom left corner of burner	58
	Center of burner	80
	Upper right corner of burner	110
Saucepan, Frying pan, Kettle	All utensils are placed in the center of preheated burner.	111 67 45
Frying pan Kettle Saucepan Saucepan Saucepan	All utensils are heated **empty** (hazard situation) during five minutes. Center of burner Bottom left corner of burner Upper right corner of burner	113 69 100 64 150

The hygrometer starts to react immediately when steam is released. The saucepan without lid carries more knowledge about boiling phenomena. The variations of the relative humidity while water is boiling are illustrated in Table 4 and in Fig. 15.

Table 4. Variations of the relative humidity while heating water in different utensils.

Utensil	%RH (begin)	%RH (boil)	%RH (after 1 min of boil)	%RH (after 2 min of boil)
Kettle	45	51	75	87
Saucepan without lid	42	88	100	100
Saucepan with lid (removed after water boils)	43	45	100	100
Saucepan with lid (not-removed)	43	45	48	50

To summarize, we tested and determined the imprecisions of the selected sensors in order to determine the corresponding thresholds that separate between risk and normal situations during cooking in a real-world environment.

Test of CO Gas Sensor. In order to test CO gas sensor, we performed the same experiments used to test VOC and Alcohol sensors during cooking. Using several types of food: fish, sausage, and heated oil (50 ml of canola oil) in a frying pan. Combustion of nutritional elements is either complete (produces Carbon dioxide CO_2) or incomplete (produces Carbon monoxide CO). Therefore, we found that when CO gas concentration in the cooking smoke reaches around 800 ppm (parts per million) then, there is an intoxication risk.

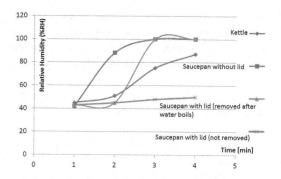

Fig. 15. Relative humidity while heating water in different utensils/configurations.

The concentration of CO in the cooking smoke was around 40 ppm for experiments illustrated in Fig. 16. So, we determined experimental threshold value of concentrations of CO gas in order to distinguish between normal and intoxication by gas/smoke risk situations during cooking.

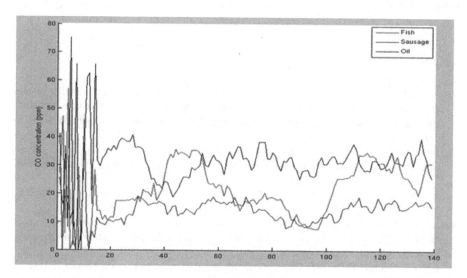

Fig. 16. Concentration of CO while cooking different food materials.

4 Conclusion

Enabling kitchen safety is a major factor for elderly people independent living. The main safety issues related to cooking are the three major risks of fire, burn (by contact or splash), and intoxication (by gas or smoke). We introduced in this paper our building of a context-aware cooking-safe system to prevent the three risks (to our knowledge this is the first study that addresses the three risks and proposes a complete system).

A result summary of our risk analysis and assessment study is presented in this paper. This study enabled us to identify the pertinent contextual parameters to monitor around oven as: concentration of VOC, Alcohol, CO gases in the cooking smoke, temperature of utensil, temperature of burner, relative humidity, and presence of utensil on burner.

We discussed in details the architecture of our system, including the hardware, the selected appropriate sensors to collect context, and a solution for sensors positioning in real-world settings.

The testing and validation activities were also discussed in this paper. As results, this testing enabled us to determine the capacity, precision and limitation of the selected sensors in real-world settings. The results also enabled us to determine the threshold values to discriminate normal from risk situations.

The presented results are the foundation of our work on building a comprehensive context-aware solution and designing algorithms to prevent risks occurring in elderly people daily living. We believe that our context-aware cooking-safe system is a block stone to enhance safety during cooking. As ongoing directions, we are working on an ergonomic evaluation of the system in order to improve the system efficiency. Furthermore, we are working on building intervention strategies that can be used when detecting risks.

References

1. Abdulrazak, B., Yared, R., Tessier, T., Mabilleau, P.: Toward pervasive computing system to enhance safety of ageing people in smart kitchen. International Conference of Information and Communication Technologies for Ageing Well and e-Health (ICT4AgeingWell'2015) (2015)
2. Abdulrazak, B., Roy, P., Gouin-Vallerand, C., Belala, Y., Giroux, S.: Micro context-awareness for autonomic pervasive computing. Int. J. Bus. Data Commun. Network. (IJBDCN) 7(2), 49–69 (2011)
3. Ahrens, M.: Home smoke alarms: the data as context for decision. Fire Technol. 44(1), 313–327 (2008)
4. Alwan, M., Dalal, S., Mack, D., Kell, S.W., Turner, B., Leachtenauer, J., Felder, R.: Impact of monitoring technology in assisted living: outcome pilot. IEEE Trans. Inf Technol. Biomed. 10, 192–198 (2006)
5. Billette, J., Janz, T.: Living Arrangements of seniors. Canadian Census, Ottawa (2011)
6. Chen, J., Chi, P., Chu, H., Chen, C., Huang, P.: A smart kitchen for nutrition-aware cooking. IEEE Pervasive Comput. 9(4), 58–65 (2010)
7. Doman, K., Kuai, C.Y., Takahashi, T., Ide, I., Murase, H.: Video cooking: towards the synthesis of multimedia cooking recipes. In: Lee, K.-T., Tsai, W.-H., Liao, H.-Y.M., Chen, T., Hsieh, J.-W., Tseng, C.-C. (eds.) MMM 2011 Part II. LNCS, vol. 6524, pp. 135–145. Springer, Heidelberg (2011)
8. Goldstein, M.: Carbon monoxide poisoning. J. Emerg. Nurs. JEN. Official Publ. Emerg. Dept. Nurses Assoc. 34(6), 538–542 (2008)
9. Hall, J.R.: Home Cooking Fire Patterns and Trends. Quincy, MA (2006). National Fire Incident Reporting System (NFIRS)

10. Jacobsen, A., Kent, M., Lee, M., Mather, M.: America's aging population. Popul. Bull. **66** (1), 1–20 (2011)
11. Loraine, A., Cole, S., Daniel, G., Wan, H.: 65 + in the United States U.S. Census Bureau. Government Printing Office, Washington DC (2014)
12. Lushaka, B., Zalok, E.: Development of a sensing device to reduce the risk from kitchen fires. Fire Technol. **50**(3), 791–803 (2014)
13. Martel, L., Menard, F.: Statistics Canada. Canadian Census, Demography Division (2011)
14. Office of the Fire Marshal. Reducing stovetop fire. Fire Marshal's Public (2009)
15. Sanchez, A., Burnell, L.: A smart home lab as a pedagogical tool. In: Peña-Ayala, A. (ed.) Intelligent and Adaptive ELS. SIST, vol. 17, pp. 293–314. Springer, Heidelberg (2013)
16. Sperling, A., Aisen, S., Beckett, A., Bennett, A., Craft, S., Fagan, M., Phelps, H.: Toward defining the preclinical stages of Alzheimer's disease: recommendations from the National Institute on Aging-Alzheimer's Association workgroups on diagnostic guidelines for Alzheimer's disease. Alzheimer. Dement. **7**(3), 280–292 (2011)
17. Toshio, O., Iwasaki, N.: Innovative applications and strategy on ICT applications for aging society: case study of Japan for silver ICT innovations. In: Proceedings of the 7th ACM International Conference on Theory and Practice of Electronic Governance (2013)
18. Wai, A.A.P., Shanthini Devi, S., Biswas, J., Panda, S.K.: Pervasive intelligence system to enable safety and assistance in kitchen for home-alone elderly. In: Abdulrazak, B., Giroux, S., Bouchard, B., Pigot, H., Mokhtari, M. (eds.) ICOST 2011. LNCS, vol. 6719, pp. 276–280. Springer, Heidelberg (2011)
19. Yahui, L., Asghar, Z., Pulii, P.: Visually-aided smart kitchen environment for senior citizens suffering from dementia. In: Proceedings of the IEEE International Joint Conference on: Awareness Science and Technology and Ubi-Media Computing (iCAST-UMEDIA) (2013)
20. Yared, R., Abdulrazak, B., Tessier, T., Mabilleau, P.: Cooking risk analysis to enhance safety of elderly people in smart kitchen. In: The 8th ACM International Conference on PErvasive Technologies Related to Assistive Environments (PETRA'2015), Greece (2015)
21. Yuan, M., Green, J.R., Goubran, R.: Thermal imaging for assisted living at home: improving kitchen safety. J. Med. Biol. Eng. **33**(4), 380–387 (2012)

Telemedicine and e-Health

Increased Engagement in Telegeriatrics Reduces Unnecessary Hospital Admissions of Nursing Home Residents

H.J. Toh[1], J. Chia[1], E. Koh[2], K. Lam[1], G.C. Magpantay[1], C.M. De Leon[1], and J.A. Low[3(✉)]

[1] GeriCare@North, AHS Programme Office, Khoo Teck Puat Hospital, Singapore, Singapore
{toh.hui.jin,chia.joanne.wk}@alexandrahealth.com.sg
[2] Ageing-In-Place, AHS Programme Office, Khoo Teck Puat Hospital, Singapore, Singapore
[3] Department of Geriatric Medicine and Palliative Care, Khoo Teck Puat Hospital, Singapore
Singapore
low.james.yh@alexandrahealth.com.sg

Abstract. Due to the lack of expert clinical involvement in the nursing homes of Singapore, frail and older nursing home residents become frequent unnecessary users of acute care services. Telegeriatrics, a pilot programme implemented by an acute hospital in Singapore used videoconferencing to provide timelier geriatric care, which could reduce transfers to the acute hospital. We assess the impact of the level of engagement with Telegeriatrics has on nursing home to hospital transfer rates. From December 2010 to March 2015, a total of 579 telemedicine consultation episodes were conducted in two nursing homes. Hospital admission rates were monitored over a 2-year period and compared against the nursing home's level of engagement with Telegeriatrics. The findings show a reduction in hospital admission rate for both nursing homes. There was a significant decrease of 33 % in hospital admission rates in the more-engaged nursing home while the less-engaged nursing home reported a 2 % increase. The results show that, by improving the availability of specialist support and with increased engagement in Telegeriatrics, unnecessary hospitalizations could be reduced. This leads to elimination of stress and disruption for the resident, as well as reduced costs and quicker medical care.

Keywords: Telemedicine · Telecommunications · Healthcare · Hospitalizations · Nursing home · Nursing home residents · Community care

1 Introduction

Older adults require unique, complex healthcare treatment which may include hospitalizations. However, a large percentage of emergency department visits and hospital admissions for people aged 65 years and above were inappropriate or treatable outside the hospital setting [1, 2].

With increasing life expectancy and low birth rates, Singapore faces the prospect of a graying citizen population and a greater prevalence of chronic diseases [3, 4]. Due to

© Springer International Publishing Switzerland 2015
M. Helfert et al. (Eds.): ICT4AgeingWell 2015, CCIS 578, pp. 81–90, 2015.
DOI: 10.1007/978-3-319-27695-3_5

frequent hospitalizations of nursing home (NH) residents, there were increased health-care costs, hospital-acquired infections, complications and morbidities. Furthermore, these hospitalizations contributed to the severe bed crunch [5]. Therefore, interventions are needed to reduce unnecessary use of acute care resources, by helping frail NH residents to recuperate in the NH.

The specialized field of geriatrics has improved diagnosis and treatment of common geriatric problems such as falls [6], urinary incontinence [7], and delirium [8]. In order to develop comprehensive care plans for frail elderly, geriatricians address also social issues like economic and demographic issues, lifestyle choices, social isolation, and caregiver stress. Assessing and considering these factors into an integrated plan of care result in reduced hospitalization rates, with some studies suggesting a reduction in medical care spending [9, 10].

Currently, care of NH residents is largely provided by the nursing staff and supplemented by occasional visits by general practitioner. Lack of geriatric specialist care in the NH has led to sub-optimal care and unnecessary transfers to hospital [11].

Videoconferencing can provide a reliable approach to remote assessment [12, 13] and tele-education [14, 15] without compromising quality.

To better organize and deliver care across different settings and strengthen partnerships to optimize use of scarce healthcare manpower, the Singapore's government strategy has been to reorganize the healthcare system into Regional Health Systems (RHS). Each RHS comprises of an acute general hospital working closely with community hospitals, nursing homes, home care and day rehab providers, as well as polyclinics and private general practitioners within the geographical region [16].

Telegeriatrics is an RHS initiative to bring care from the hospital to the NHs in the northern part of Singapore. Initiated in December 2010, Telegeriatrics helped to bridge the physical distance between the NH resident and the hospital's geriatrician, by delivering geriatric medical care to two partnering NHs via videoconferencing. The programme promotes early identification of potential medical problems in NH residents so that appropriate and timely medical interventions can be carried out. Early medical interventions can reduce incidences of acute deterioration and non-urgent use of emergency departments. In order to fulfill this aim, two main approaches are used in Telegeriatrics: telemedicine consultation and continuous nurse education and training.

Telemedicine consultation is a live, interactive video technology that allows the geriatricians to conduct their assessments entirely from a distance, with the assistance of a Telegeriatrics Nurse Training Course (TNTC)-trained nurse. TNTC is a 9-month course that aims to enhance and equip the NH nurses with specific knowledge and skills targeted at carrying out telemedicine-specific duties and managing common medical conditions, including chronic illnesses. They were also trained on how to detect and act upon signs and symptoms associated with atypical presentation in the elderly.

In alignment with the continuous nurse education and training, tele- multi-disciplinary meetings and tele- mortality audits were conducted to ensure quality and safety, and evidence-based practice.

The aim of this study was to assess if increased level of engagement with Telegeriatrics translates to lower hospital admissions.

2 Methods

2.1 Ethics Approval

Ethics approval was obtained from the National Healthcare Group Domain Specific Review Board (DSRB).

2.2 Recruitment and Setting

Over the study period from December 2010 to March 2015, two non-profit NHs agreed to participate in the study. They were recruited into the study due to existing partnership with the acute hospital.

NH1 began its partnership with the acute hospital in December 2010 while *NH2* joined in April 2012. During the study period, both NHs were not involved in any other programmes targeted at reducing residents' hospital admissions.

2.3 Telemedicine Consultation

The technology involved in this project included software, hardware, and infrastructure setups. The equipment used for carrying out two-way videoconferencing included a high-resolution camera and high-definition video monitor installed in the acute hospital and the two NHs. These equipment were mounted on a portable trolley so that telemedicine consultations can be held at different locations.

Before consultation, the TNTC-trained nurse identifies residents requiring specialist care. The nurse fills up a referral form and faxes it to the administrative assistant of the acute hospital. During consultation, the nurse presents the residents to the geriatrician, and describes presenting symptoms using the Situation-Background-Assessment-Recommendation (SBAR) technique. The geriatrician conducts basic clinical assessments on the resident with the nurse's assistance and prescribes appropriate treatment. The telemedicine consultation is documented in a telemedicine consultation form. After consultation, the form is emailed to the NH so that the nurses can follow up with the treatment plan. The form is then filed in the resident's case notes.

2.4 Continuous Nurse Training and Education

Selected registered nurses from the NHs have to undergo the TNTC to equip them with the necessary skills and knowledge before any telemedicine consultation can be conducted. The TNTC includes early identification of changes in residents' medical condition; presenting and documenting residents' case history in a systematic way; and management of basic medical conditions.

In addition, as a part of continuing nursing education, multidisciplinary meetings were held among the geriatrician, the TNTC-trained nurses, and other healthcare professionals. The purpose is to promote better care for the NH residents via discussions and knowledge-sharing on the diagnostic and treatment aspects of resident care.

In a mortality audit session, the geriatrician and the nurses review deaths of particular residents to identify modifiable risk factors and make joint decisions for improvement.

2.5   Data Collection

The hospital admission rates of two NHs were collected and compared from December 2010 to March 2015. The hospital admission rate was measured at two points: before Telegeriatrics and 3 years during Telegeriatrics. These rates were obtained from the monthly data sent by the NHs to the acute hospital. Other data including demographics, health data and consultation details were collected from the Resident Assessment form (RAF), resident case notes and telemedicine consultation form.

2.6   Statistical Analyses

Factors that affect the NH's extent of engagement with Telegeriatrics include number of scheduled and ad-hoc telemedicine consultations, multidisciplinary meetings and mortality audits. The NH that participated in more telemedicine-related activities is defined as "more-engaged", and the other NH as "less-engaged".

In examining NH residents' hospitalizations, a comparison of hospital admission rates before and during intervention was conducted. Univariate analysis was performed to assess if any statistically significant difference exist between the more-engaged and the less-engaged NH. We also examined whether the factors that influenced the level of engagement with Telegeriatrics had any impact on the NH's hospital admission rates.

Data was analyzed using SPSS version 22.0 for Windows (SPSS Inc., Chicago, IL, USA).

3   Results

579 telemedicine consultation episodes were conducted for 245 unique residents during the study period. The average consultation time per resident is 22 min (range 5–75 min). In 92 % of the consultations, the resident had multiple comorbidities. Polypharmacy was present in 35 % of the consultations. Recent history of admission (within the last 6 months) was present in 37 %. The demography of residents who have undergone telemedicine consultation is summarised in Table 1.

The average age of residents of the two NHs requiring specialist telemedicine consultations was 75 years (range 15–103), with 78 % aged 65 years and older. Their average length of stay in the NH was 35 months (range 1–275). Majority were Chinese, and belonged to the functional category III and IV. NH residents' physical, psychological, social and emotional needs are assessed using the RAF and classified into 4 functional categories from I to IV. Those in category I are the least dependent on others for care while category IV residents require total assistance and supervision for every aspect of Activities of Daily Living (ADL).

Table 2 presents the factors affecting the NH's engagement level with Telegeriatrics. *NH1* conducted more telemedicine-related activities when compared to *NH2*. Significant differences were found in factors such as the number of scheduled telemedicine consultation sessions, residents who have undergone telemedicine consultation and cases reviewed during multidisciplinary meetings.

Table 1. Demography of residents (N = 245).

Characteristic	NH1 (N = 133)	NH2 (N = 112)
Gender		
Female	89 (67 %)	46 (41 %)
Race		
Chinese	117 (86 %)	80 (71 %)
Malay	7 (5 %)	12 (11 %)
Indian	4 (3 %)	20 (18 %)
Others	5 (5 %)	0 (0 %)
Functional Category		
I	1 (1 %)	1 (1 %)
II	3 (2 %)	5 (5 %)
III	61 (46 %)	58 (51 %)
IV	68 (51 %)	48 (43 %)

Table 2. Factors affecting the level of Telegeriatrics engagement.

Factors	NH1	NH2
Scheduled consultations	130	63
Ad-hoc consultations	17	8
Residents seen at scheduled consultations	378	170
Residents seen at ad-hoc consultations	17	8
Multidisciplinary meetings	19	8
Cases reviewed during multidisciplinary meetings	39	14
Mortality audits	16	6
Cases reviewed during mortality audits	41	14

The presenting complaints that led to telemedicine consultations are presented in Table 3.

Table 3. Most common presenting complaints referred for telemedicine consultations.

NH1	NH2
Presenting Symptom (%)	Presenting Symptom (%)
Behavioural problem (32)	Behavioural problem (29)
Medication review (18)	Medication review (14)
Skin lesion/rash (8)	Skin lesion/rash (8)
Fever (6)	Oedema (7)
Poor appetite (4)	Management review (6)

The overall ranking of presenting complaints reveals that behavioural problems arising from dementia are most frequently referred for specialist consultations. This implies that behavioral problems were the most challenging to be managed independently by the nurse without a specialist input.

The next most frequently referred presenting problem by the NHs was medication review. In a study conducted in NHs in Singapore [17], there has been a high prevalence of polypharmacy and inappropriate medication use. The current practice of medication use in the NHs increases the risk of medication errors, including adverse drug reactions. Review of medication on a timely basis is therefore a good practice for the geriatricians to adopt to reduce polypharmacy [18, 19].

Skin-related problems such as rashes and cellulitis were also referred by the NHs for consultations. The other common presenting complaints were different for the two NHs. *NH1* prioritized fever and poor appetite as concerns which required specialist consultation, while the *NH2* tend to seek consultations for a follow-up review of previous management and oedema.

The most common diagnoses made by the geriatricians during telemedicine consultations are shown in Table 4.

Table 4. Most common category of primary diagnoses in telemedicine consultations.

NH1	NH2
Diagnosis Category (%)	Diagnosis Category (%)
General (31)	General (28)
Neurologic (23)	Psychiatric (19)
Skin rash (17)	Infectious (17)
Psychiatric (13)	Neurologic (12)
Neoplastic (7)	Skin rash (7)

The most common category of primary diagnoses made in telemedicine consultations for both NHs was general (mainly poor appetite, muscular pain, constipation, and nausea).

The other common diagnoses were neurologic-related (mainly vascular dementia and Alzheimer's disease), psychiatric-related (mainly depression and anxiety) and skin rash. Other conditions in the NHs were more commonly diagnosed as infectious-related (mainly cellulitis, infected wound and pressure ulcer), and neoplastic (mainly metastatic lung cancer).

The average monthly hospitalization rate for *NH1* at before Telegeriatrics (pre-intervention) was 147 per 100,000 resident-days (Fig. 1). At three years after joining Telegeriatrics, the hospitalization rate had significantly decreased by 33 % (P = 0.017). In *NH2*, a 2 % increase in hospitalization rate was observed at 3 years during Telegeriatrics (P = 0.952).

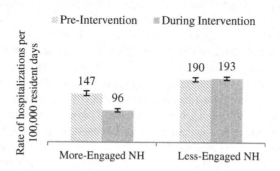

Fig. 1. Average monthly rate of hospitalizations per 100,000 resident days.

4   Discussion

NH1 is categorized as "more-engaged" as it had a higher number of telemedicine-related activities, and *NH2* as "less-engaged".

A statistically significant decrease on hospitalization rates in the more-engaged NH was observed. Similarly, in a study [11] where the more-engaged skilled nursing facilities were compared with less-engaged ones, a significant decline was found in the hospitalization rate of the more-engaged facilities. The hospitalization rate for non-engaged facilities was very similar to that of the control facilities. Hence, it is likely that if NHs were to be less engaged in the intervention, they appear to function like NHs which were never exposed to the intervention.

Telemedicine may contribute towards achieving the goal of improving clinical care. Its potential role in addressing issues arising from an ageing population, chronic conditions and rising healthcare costs has been emphasized by the European healthcare community [20]. Studies have demonstrated that the telemedicine improves quality of patient monitoring, and reduces hospitalizations and emergency department visits [21–23]. A study conducted by the U.S. Department of Veteran Affairs on 281 patients with chronic illnesses found a significant reduction in emergency department visits and hospitalizations. Furthermore, there were high levels of patient satisfaction and improved perceptions of physical health [24].

The two NHs were scheduled for a weekly consultation session and a bi-weekly session of multidisciplinary meeting and mortality audit during the study period. There was no restriction to the number of cases that can be referred to the geriatrician for each of these sessions. The less-engaged NH referred fewer cases to each session, and at several occasions, there was no telemedicine consultation session due to cancellation initiated by the NH. However, the more-engaged NH carried out consultations as per normal. The more-engaged NH was similar to the less-engaged NH, except that it had a longer time with the current administrator in place and a lower turnover of TNTC-trained nurses. Many technological programme innovators did not view technology implementation as a social process that requires personnel in following through the programme. Strong leadership and the presence of a dynamic and respected champion who encourages staff acceptance appear to have been crucial factors in the more-engaged NH. A study showed that the leading reason for successful adoption of telemedicine was that the support team had proactively identified barriers and found ways to address them [25]. The programme champions committed time and effort in garnering resources for consistent improvement and innovation, and encouraging staff adoption [26].

The results of this study must be interpreted with care because of its small sample size and lack of randomization. However, this study provided preliminary results from a comparison between a more-engaged NH and a less-engaged NH. Hence, it can be tested more rigorously with enrollment of larger, randomized and more diverse sample of NHs. Also, a control NH that did not receive telemedicine consultations or received face-to-face consultations was not included.

Also, in this study, reduced hospitalizations were regarded as the primary positive outcome of the Telegeriatrics. Other telemedicine-related outcomes such as the health-related quality of life and functional status, and resident satisfaction with care were not measured.

5   Conclusion

Telegeriatrics showed potential in reducing unnecessary hospital admissions among NH residents. The early identification of clinical issues and access to specialist support provided alternatives to the use of the emergency department. By doing so, it could contain costs while optimizing resident outcomes.

It is observed from this study that increased engagement with Telegeriatrics could be fundamental in preventing unnecessary hospitalizations. Savings from hospitalizations were only apparent in the NH that had a greater usage of telemedicine [27]. The intervention, even when made accessible to the NH, does not guarantee the NH staff's active co-operation. Telemedicine providers will have to put in further efforts to encourage engagement from the NHs. The successful adoption of technological-related interventions has been reported to be generally due to continuous support and guidance from the management [12, 28]. A team of skilled and knowledgeable NH staff who exercise teamwork is crucial to sustain the operations of using telemedicine, in order to manage current and future influences.

The next step of the study would be to measure the quality outcome indicators, in order to better comprehend the intrinsic value of support from a distance. These indicators should measure mortality, cost savings, and user satisfaction with the programme. Further research is needed to explore how the NH users perceived Telegeriatrics and the barriers that they face, which could potentially affect the NH's engagement level with Telegeriatrics.

References

1. Kim, H., et al.: Potentially preventable hospitalizations among older adults with diabetes. Am. J. Managed Care **17**(1), 419–426 (2001)
2. Wolff, J.L., et al.: Prevalence, expenditures, and complications of multiple chronic conditions in the elderly. Arch. Intern. Med. **162**, 2269–2276 (2002)
3. Cheah, J., Heng, B.H.: Implementing chronic disease management in the public healthcare sector in Singapore: the role of hospitals. World Hosp. Health Serv., **37**(3), 19–23, 40–3 (2001)
4. Cheah, J.: Chronic disease management: a Singapore perspective. BMJ **323**(7319), 990–993 (2001)
5. Tan, J.: Hospital-Acquired Infections. The New Paper, p. 7, 19 February 2013
6. Tinetti, M.E., et al.: A multifactorial intervention to reduce the risk of falling among elderly people living in the community. N. Engl. J. Med. **331**, 821–827 (1994)
7. Burgio, K.L., et al.: Behavioral vs drug treatment for urge urinary incontinence in older women: a randomized controlled trial. J. Am. Med. Assoc. **280**, 1995–2000 (1998)
8. Inouye, S.K., et al.: A multicomponent intervention to prevent delirium in hospitalized older patients. N. Engl. J. Med. **340**, 669–676 (1999)
9. Day, P., Rasmussen, P.: What is the evidence for the effectiveness of specialist geriatric services in acute, post-acute and sub-acute settings? A critical appraisal of the literature. New Zealand Health Technology (NZHTA) Report, vol. 7, no. 3, pp. 1–169 (2004)
10. Ellis, G., et al.: Comprehensive geriatric assessment for older adults admitted to hospital: metaanalysis of randomised controlled trials. BMJ **343**, d6553 (2011)
11. Ouslander, J.G.: Reducing potentially avoidable hospitalizations of nursing home residents: the INTERACT II project. Florida Medical Directors Association (FMDA) Progress Report (2009)
12. Moehr, J.R., et al.: Video conferencing-based telehealth–its implications for health promotion and health care. Methods Inf. Med. **44**(2), 334–341 (2005)
13. Casavant, D.W., et al.: Trial of telemedicine for patients on home ventilator support: feasibility, confidence in clinical management and use in medical decision-making. J. Telemedicine Telecare **20**(8), 441–449 (2014)
14. Graham, A.R.: Tele-education in medicine: why and how. Riv Med Lab – JLM **3**(1), 24–26 (2002)
15. Pedley, D., et al.: A role for tele-education in the centralization of accident and emergency services. J. Telemedicine Telecare **9**(1), 33–34 (2003)
16. Our Healthcare System, 30 October 2013. https://www.moh.gov.sg/content/moh_web/home/our_healthcare_system.html
17. Mamun, K., et al.: Polypharmacy and inappropriate medication use in Singapore nursing homes. Ann. Acad. Med. Singapore **33**(1), 49–52 (2004)

18. Finkers, F., et al.: A study of medication reviews to identify drug-related problems of polypharmacy patients in the Dutch nursing home setting. J. Clin. Pharm. Ther. **32**(5), 469–476 (2007)
19. Walsh, E.K., Cussen, K.: "Take ten minutes": a dedicated ten minute medication review reduces polypharmacy in the elderly. Ir. Med. J. **103**(8), 236–238 (2010)
20. Special issue on healthcare: healthy ageing and the future of public healthcare systems. European Commission (2009). http://ec.europa.eu/research/social-sciences/pdf/efmn-special-issue-on-healthcare_en.pdf. Accessed 22 November 2011
21. Vander Werf, M.: Ten critical steps for a successful telemedicine program. Stud. Health Technol. Inform. **104**, 60–68 (2004)
22. Smart, N.: Exercise training for heart failure patients with and without systolic dysfunction: an evidence-based analysis of how patients benefit. Cardiol. Res. Pract., **2011** (2011). Article ID: 837238. http://doi.org/10.4061/2011/837238
23. Taylor, J., et al.: Examining the use of telehealth in community nursing: identifying the factors affecting frontline staff acceptance and telehealth adoption. J. Adv. Nurs. **71**(2), 326–337 (2014)
24. McLean, S., et al.: Telehealthcare for chronic obstructive pulmonary disease. Cochrane Review and meta-analysis. Br. J. Gen. Pract. **62**(604), 739–749 (2012)
25. Ellis, D.G., et al.: A telemedicine model for emergency care in a short-term correctional facility. Telemedicine J. e-health **7**(2), 87–92 (2001)
26. Chaiyachati, K.H., et al.: Continuity in a VA Patient-Centered Medical Home Reduces Emergency Department Visits. PLoS ONE **9**(5), e96356 (2014)
27. Grabowski, D.C., O'Malley, A.J.: Use of telemedicine can reduce hospitalizations of nursing home residents and generate savings for medicare. Health Aff. (Millwood) **33**(2), 244–250 (2014)
28. Murray, E., Burns, J., May, C., Finch, T., O'Donnell, C., Wallace, P., Mair, F.: Why is it difficult to implement e-health initiatives? A qualitative study. Implementation Sci. ?: IS, **6**, 6 (2011). http://doi.org/10.1186/1748-5908-6-6

Virtual Geriatric Care: User Perception of Telegeriatrics in Nursing Homes of Singapore

H.J. Toh[1], J. Chia[1], E. Koh[2], K. Lam[1], G.C. Magpantay[1], C.M. De Leon[1], and J.A. Low[3(✉)]

[1] GeriCare@North, AHS Programme Office, Khoo Teck Puat Hospital, Singapore, Singapore
{toh.hui.jin,chia.joanne.wk}@alexandrahealth.com.sg
[2] Ageing-In-Place, AHS Programme Office, Khoo Teck Puat Hospital, Singapore, Singapore
[3] Department of Geriatric Medicine and Palliative Care, Khoo Teck Puat Hospital, Singapore, Singapore
low.james.yh@alexandrahealth.com.sg

Abstract. Older persons have unique health needs and treatment preferences that require geriatric care for comprehensive evaluation and management. Telegeriatrics was implemented in December 2010 by an acute hospital in Singapore with the aim to provide timely specialist input to nursing home residents. This preliminary study explores the perspectives of users from the NHs and the acute hospital on two aspects of Telegeriatrics – the telemedicine consultation and the nurse training programme. Seven focus group discussions and three semi-structured moderate interviews were conducted with a total of 25 participants. To identify important themes and new themes that emerged during the coding process, thematic content analysis was applied. The most commonly cited benefits were increased access to specialist care, reduced need for hospitalizations, improved quality of care, and enhanced nursing skills and knowledge. However, common perceived barriers were the lack of personal touch, technical issues, and medico-legal issues. This mode of delivering specialist care was generally acceptable to the users. To the users, Telegeriatrics showed feasibility in providing consultation, delivering education, and enhancing nursing competence.

Keywords: Telemedicine · User satisfaction · Perceptions · Healthcare · Telecommunications technology · Focus group discussion · Semi-structured interviews

1 Introduction

Telemedicine, a combination of telecommunications technology and medicine, is seen as a solution to overcome the limitations of face-to-face delivery [1–3]. In some countries, telemedicine innovations were introduced to accommodate the needs of older people in view of the ageing population [4, 5]. With an ageing population in Singapore, more old and frail people require hospitalization. As a result, Singapore's public hospitals face severe bed crunch [6, 7]. Often, hospitalization results in iatrogenic complications and declining health in the elderly [8]. Telemedicine holds potential to improving

© Springer International Publishing Switzerland 2015
M. Helfert et al. (Eds.): ICT4AgeingWell 2015, CCIS 578, pp. 91–105, 2015.
DOI: 10.1007/978-3-319-27695-3_6

outcomes for the elderly without requiring emergency department (ED) visit [9, 10]. Telemedicine consultations transcend physical limits and provide timely specialist access to the NHs. The consultations can be instrumental in detecting and treating symptoms early, thereby enabling NH residents to be managed in the NHs and preventing unnecessary transfers to the acute hospital [11–13]. Furthermore, telemedicine provides NH nurses with additional training and educational opportunities [14]. Increased access to knowledge, enhanced understanding of medical conditions and improved decision making capacity can improve the quality of care and decrease acute care transfers.

To better integrate care across different settings, the Singapore's government strategy has been to reorganize the healthcare system into Regional Health Systems (RHS). Each RHS comprises of an acute general hospital working closely with community hospitals, nursing homes, home care and day rehab providers, as well as polyclinics and private general practitioners within the geographical region [15]. Telegeriatrics is one of the RHS programmes initiated in December 2010 by an acute hospital in the north of Singapore, to provide geriatric specialist services for the elderly in three partnering NHs. Prior to the programme, limited access to specialist care resulted in heavy reliance on nursing care and physical visits by general practitioners. Limited by an inadequate supply of geriatricians, video-conferencing between the NH resident and the geriatrician enables the provision of timely care appropriate to the residents' long-term complex care needs.

One main aspect of the programme was a live telemedicine consultation with a geriatrician. A trained nurse assesses the resident at either the bedside or the consultation room, with follow-up by a geriatrician who reviews the assessment and recommends the management plan via the videoconferencing system. A high-resolution camera and high-definition video monitor were installed in the acute hospital and the NHs.

Before consultation, the nurse from the NH refers a resident requiring specialist care for consultation. In a typical telemedicine consultation, a trained nurse describes the presenting symptom(s) or problem(s), while the geriatrician identifies the root cause of the problem and prescribes the appropriate treatment. The consultation is documented in a form. This form is used to document elements of the resident's visit such as the name of consulting geriatrician, any assessments completed by the nurse and any information received from other healthcare facilities. After consultation, the form is emailed to the NH for the nurses to follow up with the management plan. Both the nurse and geriatrician play important roles in representing the effectiveness of telemedicine to provide care as this could influence user perceptions to a certain extent.

Another part of the programme was continuous education and training for the NH nurses, who are the main carers of NH residents. Before telemedicine consultations can be facilitated by the geriatrician and the nurse, selected staff and enrolled nurses from the NHs need to undergo training. The aim of the 9-month Telegeriatrics Nurse Training Course (TNTC) is to equip these nurses with a specific set of knowledge and skills targeted at managing NH residents. The nurses were also taught how to perform simple assessments and physical examinations to enable them to assist the geriatricians during telemedicine consultations. In order to ensure coordinated and integrated care, tele-multi-disciplinary meetings and tele- mortality audits were also conducted.

The acute hospital's administrators were the indirect users of Telegeriatrics as they provided the on-going support for the programme's operations. In particular, they manage matters such as administrative support, partnering NHs' feedback, and process improvements.

In several telemedicine studies, effectiveness has been explored using user satisfaction as the main outcome, and these users have reported high levels of acceptability and willingness to adopt this technology into their practices [16–18]. However, to date, these studies placed emphasis solely on usefulness of the telemedicine consultation, over general satisfaction with the programme that is required for knowledge development and quality improvement in the area of telemedicine [19, 20]. In addition, user readiness in integrating telemedicine into both clinical practice and continuous nursing education as well as the subsequent implications for patients, practices, or the wider health-care system have not been examined in the local context.

This study explores user perceptions and experience of the telemedicine system as well as the influence of education on the NH nurses in Singapore. By reporting on the users' experiences of Telegeriatrics, it is hoped that the hospital's administrators can develop targeted improvement measures to address gaps identified in the Telegeriatrics' training curriculum, processes and resources.

2 Methods

2.1 Ethics Approval

Ethics approval was obtained from the National Healthcare Group Domain Specific Review Board (DSRB).

2.2 Setting and Recruitment

Three existing NH partners of the acute hospital's Telegeriatrics programme were recruited for this study.

An interview guide was developed to elicit responses on the impact of Telegeriatrics on the quality of resident care, cost-effectiveness, user's ability to express clearly in a virtual visit, ease of equipment use, challenges, sense of intimacy, and potential for long-term use.

Staff who have used the videoconferencing system for consultations, multidisciplinary meetings and mortality audits, were included in this study.

To provide a more integrated perspective of the Telegeriatrics experience, both direct and indirect users were recruited for this study:

i. *Nurses of each NH.*
ii. *Nurse managers of each NH.*
iii. *Geriatricians of the acute hospital.*
iv. *Administrators of the acute hospital.*

The initial design of this study was to conduct only focus group discussions (FGDs) with the users. However, during its execution, we conducted three semi-structured interviews in addition to the FGDs. For one of the NHs, only one nurse manager was involved in Telegeriatrics and hence was scheduled for a semi-structured interview. A NH nurse and a geriatrician who were not available on the day of the FGD were scheduled for a semi-structured interview.

The FGDs/semi-structured interviews with the geriatricians and the hospital's administrators were held at the acute hospital while those with the nursing staff and nurse managers were conducted at the three respective NHs.

2.3   Procedures

Seven FGDs and two semi-structured interviews were conducted between February 2014 and August 2014.

Each FGD and semi-structured interview lasted approximately 1 h and 30 min respectively. The FGDs and the individual semi-structured interviews were conducted face-to-face by the first author. Prior to the FGDs and semi-structured interviews, the moderator briefed the participants on the purpose of the study, the expected duration of the session, and their responsibility as a participant in the session. They were also given sufficient time to ask questions, and signed a standardized informed consent form specifying the benefits and risks of the study. An interview guide which consisted of structured, open-ended questions was used to encourage the participants to express their unique perspectives of the programme. Field notes were taken during the sessions which allowed for triangulation of data [21] (Table 1).

Table 1. Composition of FGDs and semi-structured interviews.

Composition	Participants, N = 25
FGDs	
NH1's staff and enrolled nurses	5
NH2's staff and enrolled nurses	3
NH3's staff nurses	5
NH1's nurse managers	2
NH2's nurse managers	2
Hospital's geriatricians	2
Hospital's administrators	3
Semi-structured interviews	1
NH2's enrolled nurse	1
NH3's nurse manager	1
Hospital's geriatrician	

2.4   Data Analysis

All the FGDs and semi-structured interviews were audio recorded and were transcribed verbatim by the first author. This study used an explorative and descriptive design, in which qualitative content analysis [22] was used to search for contexts, meanings, interpretations, and consequences.

Both inductive and deductive approaches were employed in the process of the categorization. The main categories were formed mainly based on the concepts derived from literature reviews [23, 24].

The Miles and Huberman [25] framework was used for management of the data. The transcripts were first read comprehensively to obtain a general view of the main categories. They were then reviewed and coded where supplementary notes on the ideas that emerged were made, to form the main categories. The main categories were presented in a table in Microsoft Excel to allow for further thematic description, and combination of main categories and sub-categories to emerge as themes and sub-themes. Supporting comments explain these themes in the participants' own words. Identification of links and patterns between themes and sub-themes resulted.

3   Results

The study participants were mainly females, and most of which were nurses (Table 2). 76 % of the users were from the NHs, and hence the NH users' perceptions are more representative of the interview responses. All participants had no experience with facilitating consultations via the video-conferencing system before Telegeriatrics (Table 3).

Table 2. Characteristics of focus group and semi-structured interviews participants.

Characteristics	Participants, N = 25n (%)
Gender	
Female	17 (68)
Designation	
Administrator	3 (12)
Geriatrician	3 (12)
Nurse manager	5 (20)
Senior staff nurse	1 (4)
Staff nurse	9 (36)
Enrolled nurse	4 (16)

Table 3. Themes and sub-themes that emerged from FGDs and semi-structured interviews.

Themes	Sub themes
Accessibility	(i) Increased access to specialist care
	(ii) Reduced waiting and travelling time
Continuity of care	(i) Reduced need for hospital admissions
	(ii) Dying & quality of death
	(iii) Joint decision making
	(iv) Inadequacies of NHs
Impact on nursing	(i) Positive effects on nurses
	(ii) Increased expectations
	(iii) Negative impacts
Technology	(i) Receptiveness of residents'
	(ii) Technical issues
	(iii) Decreased social presence
	(iv) Personal touch
Ethics	(i) Distrust in nurses
	(ii) Medico-legal issues
	(iii) Risk of confidentiality breach

The five themes that emerged from the FGDs and semi-structured interviews were: (1) Accessibility; (2) Continuity of care; (3) Impact on nursing; (4) Technology; and (5) Ethics.

3.1 Accessibility

The users felt that the main benefit was prompt specialist attention, especially from ad-hoc consultations. This offered an opportunity for prevention and early treatment so that emergencies and hospitalizations could be prevented.

"Through telemedicine, we can start treatment straight away so [that] patients can get better... Secondly, if residents are not well, then doctor will advise sending [residents] to hospital straight away, so you administer treatment early... They also stay in hospital [for a] shorter time." **(Nurse Manager)**

The frequency of visits to the specialist clinics was also reduced, as residents did not require additional specialist medical advice after telemedicine consultations. Other cited benefits included travel expenses for specialists and hospital transfers; and reduction in stress levels associated with transferring of residents.

"Reduces doctor's travelling. Reduces the need to travel to a site, and the time involved is money." **(Geriatrician)**

3.2 Continuity of Care

Increased specialist access has resulted in managing residents on-site, therefore avoiding a trip to the ED and/or a hospital admission.

"In [the] case they (the residents) are sick, we just can call the hospital for a tele-consultation... Our admission rates are lesser now..." **(Staff Nurse)**

Better quality of death was achieved for some of the NH residents, as end-of-life care preferences were discussed during telemedicine consultations. The NH nurses could then tailor their care according to these preferences.

"They (the residents) want to die in a place where they are familiar with, with the familiar surroundings and people around them." **(Nurse Manager)**

Coordination of care through multidisciplinary meetings to address complex problems assured consistency in delivering holistic, better quality clinical care.

"I think it's very beneficial, because how can you get all the professionals together just for one case? That will be time-consuming. I think sometimes we have to maximize the use of technology." **(Nurse Manager)**

A limiting factor of continuing care in the NH was the inadequacy of resources in the NHs. This resulted in referrals to ED, even though the geriatrician and the nurse could coordinate resident care and manage conditions in the NH.

"Nursing homes have no access to equipment like [one with] diagnostic capability, for example, so to manage the patient better... Consultation alone is only one aspect." **(Nurse Manager)**

3.3 Impact on Nursing

Nurses felt a deep sense of commitment and dedication in caring for their residents. They were proud of their expanded role and appreciated that the TNTC has equipped them with confidence, knowledge, and skills. The course has also helped them to better establish information as to the nature of the problem, severity, duration and particular concerns and assess the problem's urgency. They became more alert towards any subtle changes, and knew which relevant clinician or authority to relay this information to.

"It [the TNTC] makes us, all of us, more confident, more systematic in doing assessment and delivering system of care toward the patient." **(Staff Nurse)**

In addition, the geriatricians saw the virtual consultation as a mode for the nurses to effectively deliver a concise message to the geriatrician that would result in better understanding of the resident's condition. Such skills have enabled professional growth in the nurses.

"The positive thing that you could get out of this programme would be for the nurses to be a bit sharper in their presentation, and know what our thoughts are." (**Geriatrician**)

A number of users felt that with Telegeriatrics in place, nurses must take on a more active role. For example, nurses must be able to distinguish medical conditions that require specialist care from the others, present and document accurately residents' case history, and manage more diverse conditions in the NHs.

"The tool (consultation via videoconferencing to provide care) actually forces the nurses to step up because you are trying to limit the amount of doctoring that is occurring in the nursing homes." (**Hospital's Administrator**)

A geriatrician explained that the communication skills, even when enhanced, would not be useful if the geriatricians do not have the precise questions to ask in order to elicit the information they wish to obtain from the nurse. The effort to efficiently deliver this mode of care should be shared between the geriatrician and the nurse.

"Getting them (the nurses) to do some maneuvers that are correct would be very important. The physician has to guide some of these conversations and this means, asking the right questions for the nurses or even the patient." (**Geriatrician**)

Language differences were one of the barriers to effective communication during telemedicine, affecting the quality of consultations. Language barriers were significant, particularly between foreign nurses and the local doctors.

"I still have some problems hearing the nurses properly, especially the foreign ones..." (**Geriatrician**)

Another negative impact of telemedicine was the lack of comfort and unfamiliarity with technology when the telemedicine consultations were first implemented in the NHs.

"They (the nurses) were not comfortable, having to tell the case [is] like talking to a wall." (**Nurse Manager**)

However, over time, the nurse managers observed an improvement in the nurses' confidence and competency in communication skills, and ability to facilitate consultations independently.

"They are more confident and their flair for the case presentation is much better than initially. Now they even own the whole consultation without my involvement most of the time." (**Nurse Manager**)

3.4 Technology

The nurses expressed concerns about the residents' ability to readily adopt telemedicine as a form of technology-enabled care. A nurse described how the residents exhibited initial unfamiliarity during consultations.

"Sometimes we need to repeat [our explanations] to the residents, because residents didn't know where to focus on. They didn't know about telemedicine, but they knew the doctor is with them... Sometimes they didn't know that he (the doctor) is talking to them." (**Nurse Manager**)

However, the residents were observed to adapt well to the new technology. They were receptive towards the experience and felt assured by the geriatrician's words. A nurse manager described the residents' experience as mainly positive:

"They actually acknowledge [the doctors] and they are quite happy and will wave at the doctors and they follow the instructions from the doctors." (**Nurse Manager**)

The most frequently reported challenge was the, sometimes, unfriendly medium of technology. Delays or problems with transmissions, and visual and audio quality have reportedly hindered flow of information delivery, lengthened consultation duration and made the experience a dissatisfying one.

"The reception is so poor that we have to stop because it doesn't help us at all. If we are going to have this type of reception, I say, it doesn't serve any purpose. We can't hear what is going on, we can't see [too], so it's not useful for us." (**Nurse Manager**)

Decreased social presence was also another barrier to using telemedicine. Social presence is the social degree of person-to-person awareness, which occurs in a mediated environment [26]. A geriatrician felt that the consultation affected communication due to sensory and non-verbal limitations:

"Initially, going in for [a] tele-consultation can be a bit stressful because I am not sure whether what I see and what I hear will correspond to my usual senses." (**Geriatrician**)

A common example quoted by the users was the tendency to assume that the user at the remote end could not hear them and in response, they spoke louder over the system.

"I have a habit of speaking very loudly during telemedicine. Actually they (the hospital's administrators) say I don't have to talk so loudly but then naturally, I tend to speak louder than usual." (**Geriatrician**)

The participants emphasized the importance of the geriatrician's physical presence as the doctor's touch serves as a source of comfort for the residents. Digital interaction was reported to be "different" from a physical consultation.

"There's this article about this ritual of examining the patient; it means a lot to patients. It's not necessary to listen to the lungs; you still have to put the stethoscope there." (**Geriatrician**)

"The residents are a disadvantaged group of people... Being able to have that physical connection, having that somebody to tap you on the back and say, "Hey you are okay, nothing is that wrong with you" kind of gives them that extra confidence and that boost." (**Geriatrician**)

However, they expressed understanding that although telemedicine can never replace personal touch, a key solution will be continued medical oversight. Physical visit as a follow-up to a telemedicine consultation was suggested to provide the right balance, asserting that the traditional method of face-to-face consultation should never be relinquished.

"You still need physical visits interspersed with the tele-consultation. This is to supplement the completeness, where you have one physical examination of this patient regularly..." (**Geriatrician**)

3.5   Ethics

The main ethical concern is related to trust issues between doctors and the nurses during the telemedicine consultations. Lack of trust in the nurse's ability to perform accurate physical examinations exists and this could possibly compromise the quality of resident care.

> *"There will come a time where we are so good that we don't have a clinical educator here, so the doctor there will have to really take us seriously, and whether he is going to trust that info given to him, really that decision he has to decide…"* **(Nurse Manager)**

The other potential risk associated with technology-enabled care includes potential liabilities of the health professional. With medical tele-diagnosis, medical liability is the main risk. Insecurities were expressed regarding this grey area:

> *"For some conditions, it's just not safe enough to just have telemedicine. You need to see the patient and examine the patient…"* **(Geriatrician)**

A nurse manager was concerned with the issue of patient confidentiality. With the level of details provided in multidisciplinary meetings, there was the risk that the geriatrician discusses about a resident during his meetings with other nursing homes.

> *"We have doctors going from [one] institute to [another] institute, [and] they exchange ideas… [and] then we talk about our residents… so in terms of confidentiality, I don't know how promising it is."* **(Nurse Manager)**

4   Discussion

There was a general positive response to this new way of accessing geriatric care. According to the users, the programme reduced the need for unnecessary travel and provided timely diagnosis and treatment. The users identified with the benefits of using telemedicine to manage residents remotely and improve clinical outcomes, and hence avoiding ED visits.

The nurse managers and nurses felt the benefits brought about by TNTC. Through TNTC, nurses learnt and improvised on their current nursing skills and applied them not only in telemedicine consultations, but also in their routine nursing practices. The nurse managers particularly articulated that the education aspect of the programme, including the multidisciplinary meetings, was useful, as care for the residents was coordinated among health care professionals. According to a study by Gagnon et al. [27], telemedicine applications can facilitate communication among health care professionals, and lead to a more coordinated and effective management. Also, mortality audits have helped the nurse managers and nurses assess care against standards, and identify factors that contribute to the immediate and underlying cause of death. They could address suboptimal care practices, take action to prevent such factors that could lead to similar deaths in the future, and monitor to sustain improvement. Such audits if conducted consistently and effectively have the potential to decrease morbidity and fatality, leading to standardized and improved care [28]. These after-death reviews have recently been introduced by Ministry of Health as a criterion for the enhanced set of nursing home licensing standards [29].

In addition, the nurse managers reported the success of Telegeriatrics in empowering nurses, and were keen to continue providing support needed to sustain the programme. The successful incorporation of telemedicine was reported to be mainly contributed by a supportive management that sees the need for its use [30, 31].

The nurses felt that their roles have expanded from the traditional nursing care. Prior to the programme, nurses were not expected to present cases to geriatricians nor perform physical examination on the residents during their physical visits. During the programme, increased expectations were placed on the nurses in providing resident care. Nurses were required to carry out specific tasks in the assessment and management of patients with specific conditions. Nurses were also expected to bring forth their suggestions in the management of the resident. On top of this, they had to learn how to operate the videoconferencing equipment.

Despite increased expectations, nurses expressed that they have acquired more knowledge and confidence in coordinating care. They were proud of being entrusted with this expanded role. Increased ability to partake in the care of the patient has increased nurses' engagement, as it enables greater autonomy and a voice in their working environment. Although there was initial resistance in facilitating the telemedicine consultations and frustrations with the technological disruptions, the nurses accepted these challenges. They added that this new way of delivering care has been integrated into their day-to-day nursing practice.

Nurses' attitudes toward telemedicine are the key determinant to the successful implementation of a technology-related programme [32]. Therefore, it is important to ensure that nurses are prepared to accept new operational changes, which will not only alter current medical practice but also attitudes towards a programme that involves technology. In addition, training and the presence of a support system assist the adoption and use of a new technology [33].

The geriatricians, like the nurses, regarded the increased scope of nursing care as the main positive impact of the programme. Telegeriatrics, in their perspective, was an excellent learning medium for the nurses, as it promotes sharing of clinical skills and information across the NHs.

In addition, the geriatricians felt that it was plausible to use telemedicine consultations to manage some conditions on-site. However, they appeared to be more reserved in their acceptance of the programme. They found that the care provided over telemedicine was less satisfactory than traditional encounters', as they faced difficulties in building therapeutic relationships with the residents. Similarly, complications in clinician–patient relationships created by communication technology were observed in other studies [34]. In relation to this, they and the hospital's administrators suggested that the telemedicine consultation should be a form of "relationship medicine" [35]. Telemedicine encounters should be remote only when trust between the doctor and the patient is established.

The geriatricians also felt that not seeing the patients in person and their heavy reliance on the nurses were potential medical risks. These concerns reflect a sense of insecurity in relying on a medical system that has been prone to errors [36, 37]. A study reported that the doctor took greater care in communicating with the patient in a telemedicine consultation than in a face-to-face consultation [26]. In the study, verbal cues were more frequently used to allow coordination of beliefs between both parties. Although telemedicine services have been piloted in a number of clinical domains, one of the main challenges in adopting these services includes the lack of clarity over legal liabilities [38].

The main limitation of this study is that patient satisfaction could not be assessed, as most of the NH residents were either cognitively impaired, uncommunicative or both.

Another major limitation of this study is that due to its exploratory nature, some concepts that were not mentioned in the FGDs or the semi-structured interviews were not captured in this study. Further quantitative analysis can be explored to allow a clearer understanding of the relationships among individual factors. In addition, the moderator is a member of the acute hospital team providing the telemedicine services. Hence, there is a possibility that the users may provide responses that the moderator would like to hear. In order to minimize this form of bias, an acknowledgement of participation which clarifies the process and creates a common expectation among participants was given before the discussion.

5   Conclusion

This study offers a better understanding of the ways in which Telegeriatrics had influenced the users, including its benefits and drawbacks in providing geriatric care. It identifies specific issues that can affect the user perception, and thus, it provides better guidance on how to proceed with subsequent quality improvement initiatives in order to ensure better care for NH residents.

Positive attitudes towards the programme have made it possible to coordinate treatment plans for patients on-site, and to strengthen nurses' knowledge and skills in providing better nursing care. Shared decision-making enabled the nurses to demonstrate ownership for their practice, and empowered them to manage their practice with a greater degree of professional autonomy. Telegeriatrics could be one of the solutions to compensate for the inadequate supply of geriatricians in Singapore, and play a part in the continuity of care between hospital and NHs.

While the nurses and nurse managers appreciate the programme and acknowledge that NH residents were better cared for, the geriatricians appeared to be resistant in fully embracing this programme. In many studies, the successful adoption of using telemedicine has been limited by the doctors' conservative perceptions [39, 40]. Without support of the doctors, who are central players of the programme, its operations will not be sustainable even with operational efficiency and good resource management. Hence, in order for the hospital's administrators to achieve a design that will be comfortable for the users to utilize, they need to closely assess the geriatricians' attitudes and expectations. The geriatricians must look beyond the limitations and recognize the programme's potential in providing care based in the communities which is in the best interest of patients. Also, there is a need to periodically revisit the important concept of nurse-doctor collaboration. It will require persistence, open communications, and a willingness to trust in order to overcome the nurse-doctor collaboration barriers.

The concern with the potential medical risks that comes along with the use of telemedicine highlights the need to ensure that professional practice standards are followed through and ethical standards upheld, for the protection of both the resident and the healthcare provider. The safety issues associated with telemedicine are more complicated and include not only anxiety about operating an equipment, but also concerns regarding possible adverse effects on patient management decisions through delayed or missing information, misunderstood advice, or inaccurate findings. Further research is needed in the area of patient safety as it is directly related to telemedicine practice.

The approach to success in telemedicine is to view it as a standard practice that can provide ongoing improvements in resident care. The users believed that using communication technologies to provide health care is expected, and will be more often in the near future. Telemedicine has the feasibility to extend specialist access to more areas of the community in the north of Singapore. The provision of continuous nurse education to prepare for technology use is also viable. As NH nurses play an integral part in caring for residents throughout the course of their illness, enhanced nursing knowledge and skills could potentially lead to higher standards in the provision of long-term geriatric nursing care.

Other than obtaining support from the users, it is also imperative for the programme to gain support from the health system's leadership, in order to sustain the programme's impact [41]. The remaining human, policy, and organizational issues surrounding telemedicine require attention from cross-functional research, practice, and policy teams to encourage understanding and action, in order to overcome remaining barriers that hinder the programme from achieving sustainability [41].

Acknowledgements. The authors would like to thank all the participants of this study for their time and insights.

References

1. Armstrong, I.J., Haston, W.S.: Medical decision support for remote general practitioners using telemedicine. J. Telemedicine Telecare **3**, 27–34 (1997)
2. Bashshur, R.L., et al.: Telemedicine: a new health care delivery system. Ann. Rev. Public Health **21**, 613–637 (2000)
3. Clark, R.A., et al.: Telemonitoring or structured telephone support programmes for patients with chronic heart failure: systematic review and meta-analysis. Br. Med. J. **334**, 942–945 (2007)
4. Goins, R.T., et al.: Telemedicine, rural elderly, and policy issues. J. Aging Soc. Policy **13**(4), 53–71 (2001)
5. van den Berg, N., et al.: Telemedicine and telecare for older patients–a systematic review. Maturitas **73**(2), 94–114 (2012)
6. Cheah, J., Heng, B.H.: Implementing chronic disease management in the public healthcare sector in Singapore: the role of hospitals. World Hosp. Health Serv. **37**(3), 19–23, 40–43 (2001)
7. Ong, J.: Singapore Budget 2014: Hospital bed crunch comes under fire. The Straits Times, 12 March 2014. http://www.straitstimes.com/

8. Creditor, M.C.: Hazards of hospitalization of the elderly. Ann. Intern. Med. **118**(3), 219–223 (1993)

9. Shah, M.N.: High-intensity telemedicine-enhanced acute care for older adults: an innovative healthcare delivery model. J. Am. Geriatr. Soc. **61**(11), 2000–2007 (2007)

10. Trief, P.M., et al.: Psychosocial outcomes of telemedicine case management for elderly patients with diabetes the randomized IDEATel trial. Diab. Care **30**(5), 1266–1268 (2007)

11. Ellis, D.G., et al.: A telemedicine model for emergency care in a short-term correctional facility. Telemedicine J. E Health **7**(2), 87–92 (2001)

12. McLean, S., et al.: Telehealthcare for chronic obstructive pulmonary disease: cochrane review and meta-analysis. Br. J. Gen. Pract. **62**(604), 739–749 (2012)

13. Grabowski, D.C., O'Malley, A.J.: Use of telemedicine can reduce hospitalizations of nursing home residents and generate savings for medicare. Health Aff. (Millwood) **33**(2), 244–250 (2014)

14. Janet, L.G.: The virtual clinical practicum: an innovative telehealth model for clinical nursing education. Nurs. Educ. Perspect. **32**(3), 189–194 (2011). National League for Nursing

15. Our Healthcare System, 30 October 2013. https://www.moh.gov.sg/content/moh_web/home/our_healthcare_system.html

16. Mair, F., Whitten, P.: Systematic review of studies of patient satisfaction with telemedicine. BMJ **320**(7248), 1517–1520 (2000)

17. Yip, M.P., et al.: Development of the Telemedicine Satisfaction Questionnaire to evaluate patient satisfaction with telemedicine: a preliminary study. J. Telemedicine Telecare **9**(1), 46–50 (2003)

18. Linassi, A.G., Li, P.S.R.: User satisfaction with a telemedicine amputee clinic in Saskatchewan. J. Telemedicine Telecare **11**(8), 414–418 (2005)

19. Demiris, G., et al.: Assessment of patients' acceptance of and satisfaction. J. Med. Syst. **28**(6), 575–579 (2004)

20. Whitten, P., Love, B.: Patient and provider satisfaction with the use of telemedicine: overview and rationale for cautious euthusiasm. J. Postgrad. Med. **51**, 294–300 (2005)

21. Burns, N., Grove, S.K.: The Practice of Nursing Research: Conduct, Critique, and Utilization, 4th edn. W. B. Saunders, Philadelphia (2001)

22. Hsieh, H.F., Shannon, S.E.: Three approaches to qualitative content analysis. Qual. Health Res. **15**(9), 1277–1288 (2005)

23. Dansky, K.H., et al.: Nurses' responses to telemedicine in home healthcare. J. Healthc. Inf. Manag. **13**(4), 27–38 (1999)

24. Greater Southern Area Health Service (GSAHS), 2009. User satisfaction and experience with a telemedicine service for diabetic foot disease in an Australian rural community, Devine Research Report. Available from: Greater Southern Area Health Service, December 2009

25. Miles, M.B., Huberman, A.M.: Qualitative Data Analysis: An Expanded Source Book. Sage Publications, Thousand Oaks (1994)

26. Tachakra, S., Rajani, R.: Social presence in telemedicine. J. Telemedicine Telecare **8**(4), 226–230 (2002)

27. Gagnon, M.-P., et al.: Systematic review of factors influencing the adoption of information and communication technologies by healthcare professionals. J. Med. Syst. **36**(1), 241–277 (2010)

28. Pattinson, R., et al.: Perinatal mortality audit: counting, accountability, and overcoming challenges in scaling up in low- and middle-income countries. Int. J. Gynecol. Obstet. **107**(1), 113–122 (2009)

29. Siau, M.E.: MOH unveils new standards for nursing homes, 9 January 2014. http://www.todayonline.com/singapore/moh-unveil-new-standards-nursing-home

30. Moehr, J.R., et al.: Success factors for telehealth—a case study. Int. J. Med. Inform. **75**(10–11), 755–763 (2006)

31. Murray, E., et al.: Why is it difficult to implement e-health initiatives? A qualitative study. Implementation Sci. **6**(6) (2011)

32. Gamm, L., et al.: Investigating changes in end-user satisfaction with an electronic medical record in ambulatory care settings. J. Healthc. Inf. Manag. **12**(4), 53–65 (1998)

33. Ash, J.S., et al.: A consensus statement on considerations for a successful CPOE implementation. J. Am. Med. Inf. Assoc. **10**(3), 229–234 (2003)

34. Weiner, M., Biondich, P.: The influence of information technology on patient-physician relationships. J. Gen. Intern. Med. **21**(1), 35–39 (2006)

35. Hixon, T.: Why is Telemedicine suddenly hot?, 22 October 2014. http://www.forbes.com/sites/toddhixon/2014/10/22/why-is-telemedicine-suddenly-hot/

36. Rowthorn, V., Hoffmann, D.: Legal impediments to the diffusion of telemedicine. J. Health Care Law Policy **14**, 1–54 (2001)

37. Sao, D., et al.: Chapter 20: Legal and regulatory barriers to telemedicine in the United States: Public and private approaches toward health care reform. In: Cohen I.G. (ed.) The Globalization of Health Care: Legal and Ethical Issues. Oxford University Press (2012, 2013). http://ssrn.com/abstract=2176764

38. Commission Staff Working Paper on Telemedicine (2009). http://ec.europa.eu/information_society/activities/health/docs/policy/telemedicine/telemedecineswp_sec-2009-943.pdf

39. Siwicki, B.: Telemedicine. Providing proof to payers. Health Data Manag. **5**(7), 56–58 (1997)

40. Coiera, E.: The guide to health informatics. Oxford University Press, Madison Avenue (2003)

41. LeRouge, C., et al.: Crossing the telemedicine chasm: have the U.S. barriers to widespread adoption of telemedicine been significantly reduced? Int. J. Environ. Res. Public Health **10**(12), 6472–6484 (2013)

Modeling and Predicting the Human Heart Rate During Running Exercise

Matthias Füller[✉], Ashok Meenakshi Sundaram, Melanie Ludwig,
Alexander Asteroth, and Erwin Prassler

Bonn-Rhein-Sieg University of Applied Sciences,
Grantham-Allee 20, 53757 Sankt Augustin, Germany
{matthias.fueller,alexander.asteroth,erwin.prassler}@h-brs.de,
{ashok.meenakshi,melanie.ludwig}@smail.inf.h-brs.de
http://www.inf.fh-bonn-rhein-sieg.de

Abstract. The positive influence of physical activity for people at all
life stages is well known. Exercising has a proven therapeutic effect on the
cardiovascular system and can counteract the increase of cardiovascular
diseases in our aging society. An easy and good measure of the cardiovascular feedback is the heart rate. Being able to model and predict the
response of a subject's heart rate on work load input allows the development of more advanced smart devices and analytic tools. These tools
can monitor and control the subject's activity and thus avoid overstrain
which would eliminate the positive effect on the cardiovascular system.
Current heart rate models were developed for a specific scenario and
evaluated on unique data sets only. Additionally, most of these models were tested in indoor environments, e.g. on treadmills and bicycle
ergometers. However, many people prefer to do sports in outdoors environments and use their smart phone to record their training data. In
this paper, we present an evaluation of existing heart rate models and
compare their prediction performance for indoor as well as for outdoor
running exercises. For this purpose, we investigate analytical models as
well as machine learning approaches in two training sets: one indoor exercise set recorded on a treadmill and one outdoor exercise set recorded by
a smart phone.

1 Introduction

People strive for a long, healthy, independent and self-determined life. A 2012
report of the WHO [1] shows that the average life expectancy in Europe increased
by more than five years between 1980 and 2010. While this sounds good in the
first place, the over-aging of our societies results in a higher number of so-called
societal diseases like cardiovascular problems or diabetes. These diseases will
have a negative impact on the cost for the public health system. Therefore,
aging societies will be one of the future problems, significantly influencing all
civilized nations around the world. A detailed look on the figures for health
costs shows that Europe spends more than 195 bn EUR [2] for cardiovascular
diseases. One can easily extrapolate the costs per year to deal with the effects of

© Springer International Publishing Switzerland 2015
M. Helfert et al. (Eds.): ICT4AgeingWell 2015, CCIS 578, pp. 106–125, 2015.
DOI: 10.1007/978-3-319-27695-3_7

societal diseases like e.g. cardiovascular problems, diabetes, high-blood pressure, arthrosis, obesity. Especially, the cardiovascular diseases are the main causes of death with almost 50 % in western industrial nations [3].

A key factor for healthy aging is physical activities. [4] shows that people who perform just moderate physical activity have a two times higher probability of healthy aging. However, these physical exercises need to be performed in a controlled manner to achieve maximum efficiency – and more important, especially for the elderly – to avoid negative effects on the health caused by an overstrain of the body [5,6]. Ignoring the limits of the physical capabilities will come with a high risk of overstraining the subject and will not only nullify the effect of the exercise but also reduce the motivation of the subject to perform exercises. A trainer, therapist or smart device that proposes user-specific work plans needs to understand and predict the response of the subject to a certain exercise strain. An easy to measure response index of the cardiovascular system is the heart rate (HR), which is used in many mobile applications and training devices to monitor the subject's exercise. These devices record and monitor the training and create some performance numbers based on the data. Reliable prediction models that establish a functional relation between the exposed strain to the subject and the response of their cardiovascular system are still missing.

In previous work the authors [7] evaluated the prediction performance of existing heart rate response models for running in indoor environments. The work presented in this article extends the work with a comparison of the prediction performance for outdoor running activities. The prediction performance is required in two aspects: First, it will support the automatic generation of user-specific training as indicated above. Second, a prediction of the response of the subjects's heart rate to strain is essential for smart training devices such as treadmills for indoor environments or pedelecs or mobile apps in outdoor environments. A decent prediction performance will allow smart devices to determine the right dose of strain that leads to an optimal training or therapy result.

Existing approaches to modeling the heart rate response to running exercises can be divided into two classes: (i) analytical models, which contain closed-form equations that represent a response of the heart rate to strain, and (ii) machine learning approaches, which do not encode any prior information but will try to learn and generalize the response model in the learning process. While the first class of approaches gains its appeal from its analytical closed-form notation, the second class is attractive because it also allows accounting for environmental parameters such as altitude, slope, or any other relevant information that is not represented in the analytic equations.

This article starts with a summary of the related work, followed by a detailed description of the modeling approaches used in this evaluation. Section 4 presents the performance of the models for indoor and outdoor environments. Section 5 provides a discussion and interpretation of the results. The last section concludes the evaluation and provides some future work tasks.

2   Related Work

Today's fitness devices such as GPS watches, bracelets, step counter, or smart phones[1] are widely applied for measuring a subjects's fitness and performance. These devices monitor a subject's heart rate during an exercise and inform the subject if the heart rate is above or below a given threshold. They do not influence the exercise directly, i.e. by providing some haptic feedback. All of these devices come along with a web portal that provide a visualization of a subject's training data, statistics about the training and recommend certain exercises. However, the recommendations are rather minimalistic and include only the duration of an exercise and set-point values for the heart rate.

Heart rate models that describe a subject's response to a workload have been studied for decades [8,9]. A well-known model for treadmill and ergometer control systems were presented by [10,11]. These authors introduce a nonlinear state-space model to predict the heart rate behavior of a subject based on the running velocity on a treadmill. The nonlinear components in the state-space system allows to represent changes in the organism due to long term exercises. [12] use a slight modified model to regulate the heart rate using a bicycle ergometer and present the generic application of this model to different sports activities. [13] present a second order LTI model to describe the response for cycling, walking and rowing exercises. Their model uses the exercise frequency as input and is thus generic to different activities as well. [14] uses a Hammerstein model for cycling exercises on a home trainer. Similar model-based systems for running, cycling or rowing on respective training devices can be found in [15–19].

With the use of smart phones and their sensors, new response model applications have been investigated. [20] uses accelerometer information to predict the heart rate for a specific activity up to 1 h. [21] estimates the heart rate dynamics via smart phone sensor data that are analyzed by a neural network. The environmental condition is included as a gradient factor as well. However, the proposed model is tested for walking and hiking only.

With increasing computational power, the use of machine learning techniques to model the nonlinear relation between the heart rate and its affecting factors has gained attention. Support vector regression (SVR) is used in [22] to study the nonlinear behavior of cardiovascular variables. This resulted in a nonparametric model that quantitatively describes the observations made. SVR was further used by [23] in a model-predictive control framework for regulating the intensity of the exercise. Neural network (NN) is another machine learning technique and is highly capable in modeling nonlinear pattern in the data. [24] used NNs to estimate the activity based on a given time-series of heart rate data. However, the structure and weights of the network plays a important role in the modeling and wrong weights and structure will result in a faulty model. [25] used an evolutionary technique to find a good structure and weight of the networks in the available search space to ensure a good heart rate response model.

---

[1] e.g. http://www.garmin.com, http://www.fitbit.com, http://www.polar.com, http://www.runtastic.com.

Another application of predictive heart rate models is automated training plan generation. An eHealth application presented by [26] uses the analytic model of [10] to generate optimal training protocols while avoiding an overstrain of the subject. The training protocol includes estimated running velocity but does not include environmental conditions. [27] evaluated the generic heart rate model that is capable of transferring the response of a subject between cycling and running exercises. They include their model in a training plan generation system that is capable of predicting the response of a certain training in advance.

The presented literature provides solutions and applications of heart rate response models. However, the results are hard to compare since they used different type of exercise protocols and workloads. A study presented by [28] performs a comparison of time-variant mathematical models for outdoor cycling. The results presented in this paper is one step towards the evaluation of analytical and machine learning models for indoor and outdoor exercises.

3   Modeling Approaches

In the following, we present two baseline models as a reference, and a set of analytic and machine learning models in detail that we evaluate in this work. All models predict the heart rate in beats per minute (bpm).

3.1   Baseline Models

As a reference mark for the performance of the analyzed models, we introduce the so-called *baseline models*. These models are simple and do no have any physiological meaning. The first model for prediction is a simple point shift over the specified time horizon. This model is the reference for the prediction over all evaluated horizons up to 120 s. The second one is a polynomial model to simulate an entire training session. The polynomial model does not have any feedback and thus does not allow to update the modeling using measured heart rate.

– **Pointshift Model:** The modeled heart rate is produced as the measured heart rate with a time shift according to the defined time horizon. To predict w seconds, we call w the *winsize* and model the heart rate y at each point of time t as $y(t + w) = hr(t)$ where hr is the measured heart rate. The model stops when the training is finished. Any kind of workload is completely ignored in this case.

– **Polynomial Model:** The modeled heart rate is given by the quadratic polynomial $y(t) = a_0 + a_1 \cdot u(t) + a_2 \cdot u^2(t)$ with three parameters $a_0, a_1, a_2 \in \mathbb{R}$ and velocity u. This model is just a scaling function as easy as possible for mapping any kind of input data (like workload) to any kind of output data (like heart rate). We used this function as baseline function to determine the fitting-quality without any physiological modeling.

3.2 Analytical Models

For all analytical models presented here, the input signal $u(t)$ is the velocity imposed to the runner. The model output is a prediction of the heart rate. The specific model parameters were identified by using a recursive least square algorithm (Levenberg-Marquardt) for minimizing the error as recommended in [29]. The ODE system are solved using an explicit runge-kutta method of order 5 due to Dormand & Prince [30]. In this research, we analyzed the following analytic models:

- **ODE Model by Cheng et al.** [10]: The differential equation model from Cheng et al. is originally used for treadmill walking and is described as follows:

$$\dot{x}_1 = -a_1 x_1(t) + x_2(t) + g(u(t))$$
$$\dot{x}_2 = -a_4(x_2(t) - \tanh(x_2(t))) + a_5 x_1(t)$$
$$g(u(t)) = \frac{a_2 u^2(t)}{1 + \exp(-u(t) + a_3)}$$
$$y(t) = HR_{rest} + x_1(t)$$

  The model is initialized with $x(0) = [x_1(0) \quad x_2(0)]' = [0 \quad 0]'$. The change in heart rate from the resting heart rate (HR_{rest}) is represented by x_1, whereas x_2 is a non-measurable variable to simulate the slow reaction of human metabolism in dependency of x_1 like effects from hormonal system, increase in body temperature or other slow-acting effects. The nonlinear function $g(u(t))$ models the non-linear behavior of the heart rate to workload. The model uses five parameters $a_1, \ldots, a_5 \in \mathbb{R}^+$.

- **ODE Model by Paradiso et al.** [12]: The differential equation model from Paradiso et al. is originally used for cycling. The second-order time-invariant nonlinear system is described as

$$\dot{x}_1(t) = -a_1 x_1(t) + a_2 x_2(t) + a_6 u^2(t)$$
$$\dot{x}_2(t) = -a_3 x_2(t) + a_4 f_{a_5}(x_1(t))$$
$$f_{a_5}(x_1(t)) = x_1(t) \cdot \frac{1}{1 + e^{-x_1(t) - a_5}}$$
$$y(t) = HR_{rest} + x_1(t)$$

  where f_{a_5} is a Lipschitz continuous function in dependency of a_5. This is used to model the non-linear behavior of the heart rate to workload. The $x_1(t)$ describes the changes in heart rate from resting heart rate. Similarly to the previous model of Cheng et al. x_2 models the slow-acting effects of the metabolism. The model uses six parameters $a_1, \ldots, a_6 \in \mathbb{R}^+$.

- **LTI Model** [13]: The second order linear time invariant model as below is originally used for heart rate prediction during walking, cycling and rowing exercise:

$$y(t) = a_1 \cdot y(t-1) + a_2 \cdot y(t-2)$$
$$+ a_3 \cdot u(t-1) + a_4 \cdot u(t-2)$$

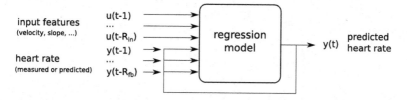

Fig. 1. Machine learning model with different numbers of input and feedback regressors.

where $y(t) = \Delta HR(t)$ is the measured change in heart rate at time t. The model uses four parameters $a_1, \ldots, a_4 \in \mathbb{R}$. It is mentioned in [13] that the second order model is the optimal dimension, higher order models do not improve the performance.

– **Takagi-Sugeno Model (TS)** [14]: This is a modified Hammerstein model and is originally used for controlling a cyclic ergometer for elderly non-trained people.

$$x(t+1) = (Ax)(t) + \sum_{i=1}^{2} h_i(u(t))B_i u(t) + B_{u0}$$

$$y(t+1) = x_1(t+1)$$

with

$$h_1(u(t)) = \frac{u(t) - u_{\min}}{u_{\max} - u_{\min}}, \quad h_2(u(t)) = \frac{u_{\max} - u(t)}{u_{\max} - u_{\min}},$$

and $B_1 = B_{u1} + u_{\max}B_{u2}$, $B_2 = B_{u1} + u_{\min}B_{u2}$ and

$$A = \begin{pmatrix} a_1 & 1 & 0 \\ a_2 & 0 & 1 \\ a_3 & 0 & 0 \end{pmatrix}, \quad B_{ui} = \begin{pmatrix} \gamma_{0i} \\ \gamma_{1i} \\ \gamma_{2i} \end{pmatrix}.$$

x is the n-size state ($\mathbb{R}^3$) of the system. The first element in x represents the heart rate of the subject. The others are set to zero at the beginning of each exercise. The model has twelve parameters $a_i, \gamma_{0i}, \gamma_{1i}, \gamma_{2i} \in \mathbb{R}, i \in \{1, 2, 3\}$.

3.3   Machine Learning Models

We present three common machine learning approaches that can be used for heart rate modeling and prediction during a running exercise. These approaches can further be categorized by their input and feedback signals dimensions, called regressors. Figure 1 sketches the possible differences. By using an input regressor dimension of 1, the model uses the input signal of the current time (denoted by $R_{in} = 1$). By increasing the regressor dimension, the model can make use of past input values that may influence the upcoming heart rate. A regressor value of, e.g. $R_{in} = 6$ means that the model uses the last six input values. In our example

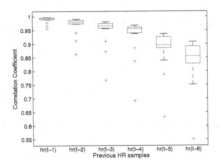

Fig. 2. Correlation of current heart rate sample with six previous heart rate samples.

with 10 s sampling rate, the model input covers the last 60 s. The same regression can be applied to the feedback signal. A feedback signal of e.g. three ($R_{fb} = 3$) uses the last three heart rate values to predict the upcoming one. The one step prediction can be applied further steps ahead by feeding the model output back into the feedback input. This allows to predict or simulate the system infinite steps ahead. The drawback of the feedback approach is that multi-step prediction relies on previous predictions, and thus the errors may accumulate.

The input features for the learning approaches in this work consists of the running velocity, distance run and the estimated slope based on the altitude changes. We further use different size of feedback regressors to evaluate the influence on these. The notion of using previous heart rate samples to predict current heart rate was discussed in [25]. The current heart rate has a linear correlation with the immediately preceding heart rates. Figure 2 shows the correlation between the six previous instances of the heart rate to the current heart rate in the data set. Based on the prediction performance, feature dimensionality and distinct information provided by the features, we chose to evaluate the prediction performance by providing different heart rate feedback i.e. no heart rate feedback until six heart rate feedback. The results are shown in the later section. As a preprocessing step in all approaches, we standardize the data to have zero mean and unit variance.

– **Linear Regression** (LR) [31] is a statistical technique used to model the input and output variable relationship. This relation is established by a linear predictor function which consists of a linear combination of explanatory variables to produce the output response variable.

$$\hat{y}(w, x) = w_0 + w_1 x_1 + \cdots + w_p x_p$$

$\hat{y}$ is the response variable, $x = (x_1, \ldots, x_p)$ are the explanatory variables, p is the number of explanatory variables, $w = (w_1, \ldots, w_p)$ are the unknown coefficients and w_0 is the intercept. For heart rate modeling and prediction, the features described earlier will be the explanatory variables and the heart rate to be predicted is the response variable. Using the least square algorithm to minimize the residual sum of squares between the observed and predicted responses, the unknown coefficients and intercept are calculated. Detailed study on linear regression approach can be found, for example, in [32]. Linear regression for heart rate prediction is also studied in [33].

– **Multilayer Perceptron** (MLP) [34] is an artificial feedforward neural network used to relate input variables to the corresponding output variables. A feedforward MLP has an input layer, a number of hidden layers and an output layer. The number of hidden layers and the mode of connection between each layer can be also varied depending on the application. In our approach to model heart rate, the network has two hidden layer with sigmoid activation function and the nodes in each layer are fully connected to the nodes in the subsequent next layer. A bias is also attached to hidden and output layers. Supervised learning techniques are used to learn the weights of the links that connect the nodes in each layer. In this case, backpropagation along with gradient descent is used to learn the weights. Mathematically, the following equation describes each non-input layer in the artificial neural network:

$$y = \varphi(w^T x + b)$$

where y is the output to the next layer, x is the input vector i.e. output from the previous layer, w is the weight vector, b is the bias and φ is the activation function. In order to avoid local minima, training is done in multiple epochs. To approximate the true output value with a accuracy comparable to the other models, it takes the network about 500 training epochs with 25 % of the training data used for cross validation. By trial and error, the learning rate and learning rate decay are found to be 0.001 and 1.0 respectively. The selection of the learning rate and other learning parameters has a huge influence on the resulting performance of the MLP model. One future task is to identify an optimal set of parameters and the network structure by conducting a detailed study on the influence of each of these to the prediction performance. During training, the features described earlier act as the input and the recorded heart rate available in the data set is the output. For testing, the same features act as input and the output heart rate is predicted. Neural networks for heart rate prediction are also discussed in [21, 25].

– **Support Vector Regression** (SVR) is based on Vapnik-Chervoenkis theory introduced in [35]. The goal is to find a function $f(x) = w \cdot \phi(x) + b$ that remains as flat as possible and has at most ϵ deviation from actual targets. Let $\{(x_1, y_1) \ldots (x_n, y_n)\} \subset \chi \times \mathbb{R}$ be the given training data where χ is the input space or the dimension of the input features. The high dimensional x is nonlinearly transformed using an appropriate kernel function $\phi(x)$ to a lower dimension. The kernel function in this case is considered to be radial basis function. The coefficients w and b are identified by minimizing a regularized risk function with the allowed ϵ deviation. The regularization constant and ϵ can be varied depending on the application. The selection of these values could impact the prediction performance by over or under fitting the given training data. But it is not practical to search a very large space for all combinations of these values. Therefore, a grid search over a possible set of values for each parameter combined with k-fold cross validation technique is performed. The best parameter set with minimal average mean squared error is found and used thereafter. During training, the features described earlier act as the input and the recorded heart rate available in the data set is the output. For testing, the same features act as input and the output heart rate is predicted. Tutorials on SVR can be found in [36]. Use of SVR for cardiovascular systems can also be found in [22,33].

4   Results

The following section evaluates the analytic and machine learning models discussed earlier. The performance is evaluated based on the mean squared error (MSE in bpm^2) between the measured heart rate and the predicted one for a certain time horizon based on the current input data. This multi-step prediction is needed, for example, to properly control the strain imposed to the subject by a smart training device. The model should predict if the heart rate increases or decreases and thus allows the controller to reduce or increase the workload on the subject in time. The time horizon (w) for this analysis was chosen to 10, 20, 30, 60, 90 and 120 s. For all models with a feedback loop (analytic as well as machine learning), we simulated the response of the subject while updating the feedback using the measured heart rate up to time t. For time t to $t+w$, we simulate the system and close the loop from the output back to the feedback input. A complete simulation of a training session in needed for an automatic generation of training plans. The generator is able to predict the heart rate response for a specific plan and can improve the plan by the use of the model response of the complete training session. The session simulation is marked with ∞ in the prediction horizon.

The first part of the evaluation starts with the indoor exercises on the treadmill. Since all of the presented models were developed for indoor environments, the indoor performance can be seen as the maximum performance of the model. The second part of this section evaluates the same models for outdoor running exercises. Each set of indoor and outdoor training sessions were used in a leave-one-out cross validation where $n-1$ data sets were used for identifying the model parameters and the evaluation is performed for the remaining session. This was repeated combinatorially to have each session evaluated once.

4.1   Indoor

Experimental Setup. The experimental data for these indoor and outdoor experiments were recorded from a 30 years old subject (male, BMI of 21). The resting heart rate is identified in the resting phase before every session. To cover many aspects of the heart rate response of the subject, the three different types of exercises were performed.

1. **A Simple Onset/Offset Exercise.** The exercise includes one single velocity at 7 km/h for 15 min. This protocol is a basic exercise at a velocity usually used for endurance training.

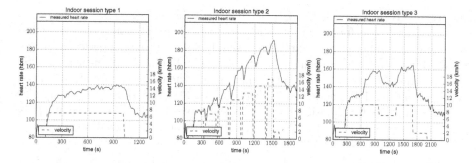

Fig. 3. Example data set for indoor exercise type 1, 2 and 3.

2. **A Step Exercise Protocol.** The protocol starts with 5 km/h and increases every 3 min by 2 km/h until the subject is exhausted. This step protocol provides a range from nearly walking velocity up to maximum velocity and thus provides the complete heart rate response between resting heart rate and maximum heart rate. The protocol was performed for a performance diagnostic of the subject. There is a 30 s pause after every step to take lactate samples. The results of this performance test is not relevant for this work. The pauses between each step provide information about the recovery of the heart rate.

3. **An Interval Protocol.** The protocol has two alternating velocities. The exercise starts with 7 km/h for 6 min, followed by a 10 km/h phase for 6 min and repeating again 7 km/h and 10 km/h for 6 min each. This type of protocol provides some information about the recovery and fatigue of the subject while running at two alternating velocities.

All indoor exercise protocols include a recovering phase after the end of the exercise to provide information about the recovery behavior of the subject. In the recovery phase, the subject still walks 5 min at 2 km/h to relieve the cardiovascular system of the subject. Figure 3 shows the indoor exercise protocol and an example of the subject's heart rate for each type.

The indoor experiments were performed on a Woodway[2] PPS 55 med treadmill. The slope of the treadmill was set to 1.5 % in all protocols. The heart beat of the subject was recorded by a Polar[3] H7 bluetooth sensor. Both systems were connected to one single data logger that record the following performance data: time (seconds), distance (meters), velocity (m/s), slope (1.5 %, static), heart rate (beats per minute). The data were sampled every second and later down sampled to 10 s interval. All in all, three of each exercise types were recorded, resulting in a complete set of nine sessions. These sessions are the input for the model identification in the indoor scenario.

---

[2] http://www.woodway.de.
[3] http://www.polar.com.

Analytic Models. Table 1 shows the average MSE (in bpm^2) for the baseline, analytical as well as for the machine learning models for all nine indoor sessions. As seen in the upper part of Table 1, the simple pointshift model performs better for short horizons up to 20 s than the analytic LTI, ODE and Takagi-Sugeno (TS) models. The LTI model has a good prediction performance compared to the more complex ODE and TS models for horizons up to 90 s. The Takagi-Sugeno model is worse for a small prediction horizon but improves for longer time spans. It is the best analytic model for a complete session prediction (simulation).

Machine Learning Models. The presented machine learning approaches LR, SVR and MLP were trained for a single-step prediction. A multi-step prediction and simulation of a complete training session is done by feeding back the predicted heart rate values in the respective input. The results of these analysis is shown in the lower part of Table 1. The numbers of input regressors and feedback regressors for each model type is denoted by $R_{in} = n$ and $R_{fb} = n$ in each line of the respective model. The machine learning have a better prediction performance than the pointshift reference for all covered time spans. The performance of LR, SVR and MLP is compareable for prediction horizons up to 30 s. For longer prediction time, SVR performs better. The simulation performance of LR and MLP are in the same range of about 50 to 60 bpm^2. The SVR performs best with a simulation performance of about 30 bpm^2.

4.2   Outdoor

Experimental Setup. The results of the indoor experiments showed that the models are able to predict and simulate the heart rate response to a certain extend. Since most of the people prefer outdoor exercise, the following experiments evaluate the performance of these models in outdoor running. The outdoor experiments do not follow any defined exercise protocol since it is hard to follow a velocity based protocol in outdoor environments. The subject was asked to perform a usual training session as one would do in the leisure time. The training session were recorded via a smart phone. The heart beat of the subject was recorded by the same Polar H7 bluetooth sensor as in the indoor experiments. The smart phone uses the heart beat sensor and its internal sensors to record the following data: time (s), velocity (m/s), air pressure (hPa), position (latitude, longitude) and the heart rate (hbm) with a recording rate of 1 Hz. The air pressure data is later used to estimate the altitude and its change based on the barometric formula and calibrated at the beginning of each session.

Figure 4 shows two example outdoor sessions. The left one is a session with only a little change of the altitude. It is a running track around a lake with one bridge in between that need to be crossed (at time 550s). The right figure shows a track with a hilly environment. It is a round course with a distance of about 1 km. The round track was run for three times. The resulting measurements of velocity, height and distance are noisy and inaccurate compared the indoor data. However, the goal of these experiments is to test the capabilities of these models in outdoor environments using standard equipment.

Table 1. Indoor results for analytical and machine learning models in MSE (bpm^2). The MSE represents the test set average over all sessions. The prediction horizon is evaluated from 10 s up to 120 s. ∞ means a simulation of the training session. For the machine learning methods, R_{in} = n means the number of input regressors and the number of feedback regressors.

	Prediction horizon (s)						
	10	20	30	60	90	120	∞
Reference models							
Polynomial	–	–	–	–	–	–	223.5
Pointshift	4.4	12.9	26.2	62.3	108.2	157.7	–
Analytical models							
LTI	8.9	13.1	17.1	27.9	38.5	48.0	82.7
ODE Cheng	14.8	16.2	31.7	59.3	74.8	84.2	110.1
ODE Paradiso	22.4	22.4	48.3	91.7	109.6	119.1	150.1
Takagi-Sugeno	12.5	17.2	23.1	30.4	36.5	43.8	52.6
Machine learning							
Linear regression							
LR ($R_{in} = 1$, $R_{fb} = 0$)	–	–	–	–	–	–	141.6
LR ($R_{in} = 1$, $R_{fb} = 1$)	3.5	8.3	12.5	23.1	32.1	46.9	58.7
LR ($R_{in} = 1$, $R_{fb} = 3$)	3.4	9.1	12.3	23.0	31.9	39.0	58.0
LR ($R_{in} = 1$, $R_{fb} = 6$)	3.4	8.1	12.3	22.5	31.0	38.2	58.5
LR ($R_{in} = 3$, $R_{fb} = 1$)	2.7	6.1	9.0	17.3	24.9	30.9	46.2
LR ($R_{in} = 3$, $R_{fb} = 3$)	3.2	8.2	12.7	24.6	34.4	41.5	56.4
LR ($R_{in} = 6$, $R_{fb} = 1$)	2.6	5.5	7.8	14.2	20.3	25.9	47.0
LR ($R_{in} = 6$, $R_{fb} = 6$)	3.2	7.7	11.8	22.5	31.8	39.3	61.6
Support vector regression							
SVR ($R_{in} = 1$, $R_{fb} = 0$)	–	–	–	–	–	–	176.2
SVR ($R_{in} = 1$, $R_{fb} = 1$)	3.0	6.5	9.2	15.4	20.4	24.4	33.0
SVR ($R_{in} = 1$, $R_{fb} = 3$)	2.9	6.3	9.0	15.1	21.8	24.0	31.6
SVR ($R_{in} = 1$, $R_{fb} = 6$)	2.9	6.3	8.7	13.9	18.1	21.5	29.1
SVR ($R_{in} = 3$, $R_{fb} = 1$)	2.6	5.4	7.5	12.7	16.8	19.9	26.3
SVR ($R_{in} = 3$, $R_{fb} = 3$)	3.0	6.3	8.5	14.0	18.3	21.6	27.8
SVR ($R_{in} = 6$, $R_{fb} = 1$)	2.5	5.0	6.5	10.2	12.9	15.0	21.6
SVR ($R_{in} = 6$, $R_{fb} = 6$)	2.9	5.4	6.7	9.6	12.2	14.3	20.3
Multi layer perceptron							
MLP ($R_{in} = 1$, $R_{fb} = 0$)	–	–	–	–	–	–	325.0
MLP ($R_{in} = 1$, $R_{fb} = 1$)	6.2	14.8	22.2	36.6	45.7	51.3	62.2
MLP ($R_{in} = 1$, $R_{fb} = 3$)	3.9	8.7	12.6	21.1	27.7	33.9	56.1
MLP ($R_{in} = 1$, $R_{fb} = 6$)	3.8	7.8	10.7	19.8	30.0	39.0	66.5
MLP ($R_{in} = 3$, $R_{fb} = 1$)	3.5	7.4	10.9	21.2	30.3	37.5	55.4
MLP ($R_{in} = 3$, $R_{fb} = 3$)	3.4	7.4	9.7	18.4	24.8	29.3	44.9
MLP ($R_{in} = 6$, $R_{fb} = 1$)	0.6	21.3	30.5	44.1	47.7	48.7	53.5
MLP ($R_{in} = 6$, $R_{fb} = 6$)	3.4	7.2	9.0	12.9	16.3	19.0	41.9

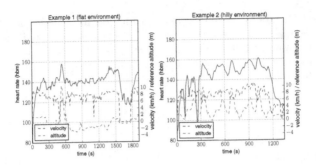

Fig. 4. Example data set for an outdoor exercise.

Analytical Models. The upper part of Table 2 shows the average MSE (in bpm^2) for the baseline and analytical models for all eight outdoor sessions. The performance of all models drop significantly compared to the indoor results. The pointshift reference models performs better for predictions up to 20 s than any analytical model. The prediction performance of LTI, ODE Cheng et al. and Takagi-Sugeno is similar for horizons between 10 and 90 s. However, the ODE model of Paradiso et al. has a better prediction performance between 60 and 120 s horizon. The Takagi-Sugeno model is again worst for short prediction horizons but it is the best analytical model for a simulation of the heart rate response for a complete training session. Overall, the simulation performance is very similar in all analytic models.

Machine Learning Models. For the machine learning approach, only the relevant regression dimensions for LR, SVR and MLP which showed a good performance in the indoor evaluation are listed in the lower part of Table 2. The other regression dimensions were tested as well, but shows a similar performance as the listed ones. The prediction capabilities of all machine learning models is similar for outdoor running. Their performance up to 120 s it better compared to the performance of the analytical models and the pointshift models. It can be seen from the figures in Table 2, that the simulation performance of LR and SVR is on the same level as the analytic approaches. While the prediction performance of MLP up to 120 s is comparable to LR and SVR, the simulation performance is worse.

5   Interpretation of Results

Indoor. The cardiovascular system has a typical delay of 60 s on an increase or decrease of the workload. For this 60 s time horizon, the LTI (MSE = 27.9 bpm^2), ODE model of Paradiso et al. (MSE = 25.9 bpm^2), Takagi-Sugeno (MSE = 30.4 bpm^2), linear regression (MSE = 23.1 bpm^2) and multi layer perceptron (MLP = 35 bpm^2) have a similar performance. Figure 5 shows the 60 s prediction and simulation performance of one example indoor session of type 3. The top left

Table 2. Outdoor results for analytical and machine learning models in MSE (bpm^2). The MSE represents the test set avarage over all sessions. The prediction horizon is evaluated from 10 s up to 120 s. ∞ means a simulation of the training session. For the machine learning methods, R_{in} = n means the number of input regressors and R_{fb} = n the number of feedback.

	Prediction horizon (s)						
	10	20	30	60	90	120	∞
Reference models							
Polynomial	–	–	–	–	–	–	203.5
Pointshift	14.7	37.3	59.1	107.3	145.6	191.1	–
Analytical models							
LTI	44.9	49.4	75.2	97.7	158.3	160.9	181.9
ODE Cheng	24.4	39.5	62.8	103.2	126.4	141.9	190.1
ODE Paradiso	21.9	35.3	51.5	74.0	88.0	99.2	185.2
Takagi-Sugeno	34.7	39.7	51.5	85.8	115.5	143.5	173.7
Machine learning							
Linear regression							
LR ($R_{in} = 1, R_{fb} = 1$)	13.2	31.0	45.3	67.3	81.6	99.0	175.1
LR ($R_{in} = 6, R_{fb} = 1$)	13.0	30.0	43.1	61.4	73.0	88.9	188.2
Support vector regression							
SVR ($R_{in} = 1, R_{fb} = 1$)	12.3	27.4	38.9	58.4	74.8	92.2	180.5
SVR ($R_{in} = 6, R_{fb} = 1$)	13.0	30.0	43.1	61.4	73.0	88.9	188.2
SVR ($R_{in} = 6, R_{fb} = 6$)	29.4	42.6	61.4	74.9	90.6	110.3	184.4
Multi layer perceptron							
MLP ($R_{in} = 1, R_{fb} = 1$)	13.3	31.2	46.0	73.5	94.9	117.3	224.0
MLP ($R_{in} = 6, R_{fb} = 1$)	14.3	32.9	47.8	73.4	92.0	110.2	363.1
MLP ($R_{in} = 6, R_{fb} = 6$)	15.9	33.5	47.8	67.3	82.2	98.3	249.3

plot shows the baseline performance of the polynomial and pointshift method. The results of the analytic and machine learning approaches are shown in the other subplots. The LTI and ODE model of Cheng et al. do underestimate the response of the heart rate at the beginning of the session whereas the Takagi-Sugeno model shows a better response behaviour. Furthermore, both approaches simulate the drop of the heart rate in the recovery phase quite well. The LR and MLP approaches show a similar underestimation of the heart rate response at the beginning of the session. MLP does not represent the recovery phase quite well. SVR method model the initial response of the session best.

A closer look on the regressor number for the linear regression models shows that the increase of input regressors has a slight positive effect on the results. However, increasing the number of feedback regressors decreases the performance of the model. A closer look in the resulting LR regression coefficients shows that

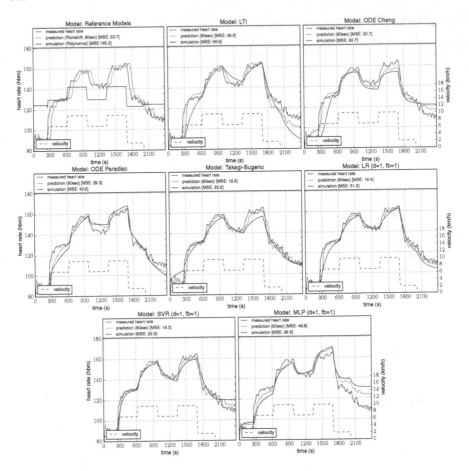

Fig. 5. Example indoor session (type 3) and prediction and simulation performance of the evaluated models. The MSE of each prediction is given in the legend of each plot.

the main weight is given to the $t-1$ regressor whereas the others are almost zero and therefore have no huge influence on the results. The support vector regression method seems to represent the nonlinearity of the heart rate response better than the linear regression method. Furthermore, the SVR method can make use of additional input regressors and perform better when more input regressors are available. An increase in feedback regressors does not have much influence. For the multi layer perceptron approach one can observe that the evaluated regressors have nearly same performance. However, a slight increase in performance can be observed at higher number of regressors.

The best performance could be achieved with the support vector regression method with a MSE of about $10\,\mathrm{bpm}^2$ for 60 s horizons and about $20\,\mathrm{bpm}^2$ for a session simulation. It has to be mentioned that the results of the SVR method are strongly dependent on the used SVR parameter for identifying the support

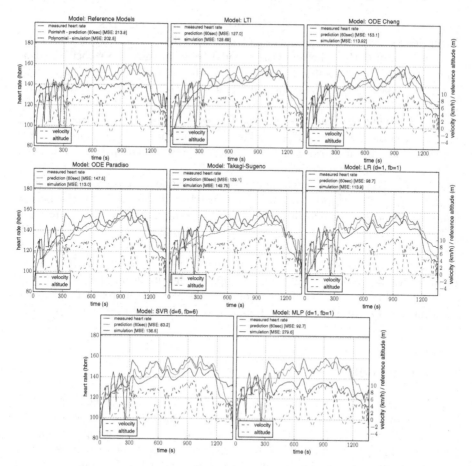

Fig. 6. Example outdoor session and prediction and simulation performance of the evaluated models. The MSE of each prediction is given in the legend of each plot.

vectors. A change in the configuration lead to a much worse performance. The prediction performance of a multi layer perceptron is compareable to the LR and SVR approaches with about 20 bpm^2.

However, the simulation performance is worse (50 bpm^2). MLP showed almost no performance change on different numbers of regressors.

Outdoor. The outdoor running exercises are not that smooth and constant as the training sessions on treadmill for the indoor evaluation. There is a high change in the workload during running caused by a fluctuation of running velocity of the subject and changes of the environment e.g., running uphill or downhill. Furthermore, the running velocity can not be recorded as accurate as for the indoor exercises since a standard smart phone with a GPS sensor was used. It can not be answered if the drop in performance is due to the high changes in velocity while performing outdoor running or due to the lower quality of the recorded data. Figure 6 visualizes the performance of the models for one example outdoor session. A look at the plot of both ODE models (time t ≈ 300 s) shows an example that the analytical models only include the velocity and no other information. The subject is running uphill and the velocity is decreasing. The actual heart rate of the subject increases due to the higher workload when running uphill. The ODE models predict a decrease of the heart rate due to the lower velocity. The charateristic can be seen several times in the plot (e.g. time t ≈ 700 or t ≈ 1000). The machine learning approaches can make use of their additional input features and thus perform better in 60 s prediction horizon compared to the analytical models.

All in all, the prediction performance of the machine learning approach is better than the analytic model approaches. It needs to be evaluated if the performance is sufficient enough for using the models in a predictive control framework.

However, the performance of the machine learning approaches LR and SVR in simulating a complete training session is in the same range as the analytical approaches ($\approx$180 bpm^2). The MLP approach shows a significant increase in the MSE in a range between 224 and 363 bpm^2. The simulation performance for outdoor training sessions is quite low compared to the indoor treadmill exercises. The simulation results are not good enough to perform an automated planning of training.

6   Conclusion

This article presented an evaluation for modeling the cardiovascular response for indoor and outdoor running activities. We distinguished the models between analytical models found in literature and machine learning models using well applied machine learning techniques like linear regression, support vector regression and multi layer perceptrons. The results were presented with different prediction horizons between 10 and 120 s as well as for a complete simulation of a training session.

The prediction performance of the analytical models for indoor running is in the range of 30 bpm^2(MSE) for a prediction horizon of 60 s and about 70 bpm^2 for the simulation. The performance of machine learning techniques shows a dependency on the used regressor size for input and feedback channels for SVR and MLP techniques but does not influence the LR models. The 60 s prediction performance for indoor running is in the range of 15–20 bpm^2 and about 40 bpm^2 for the simulation of the session with the SVR method.

A usual training zone for aerobic and anaerobic training is usually 15 to 20 bpm wide (10 % of the maximum heart rate). The best simulation performance with a mean error of 6–7 bpm (40 bpm^2) is still not sufficient enough for a detailed training plan which would require an accuracy of about 5 % of the maximum heart rate ($<$25 bpm^2)

As expected, the prediction performance for outdoor sessions is lower compared to indoor sessions. The prediction performance of the analytical models for a 60 s horizon is in the range of 90 bpm^2. The simulation performance of the analytical models for an outdoor session is about 180 bpm^2. The machine learning models shows a better performance than the analytical models for a certain prediction horizon. For these models, MSE for a 60 s prediction is about 60 bpm^2. However, the learning approaches do not provide a better simulation performance than the analytical models. LR and SVR have a similar MSE of about 180 bpm^2 while MLP has an MSE of 240 to 360 bpm^2.

The next step in our research is to evaluate more input features that have an influence on the prediction capabilities. Environmental parameters like the road condition (e.g., tar or gravel), temperature or an improved slope estimation are example features that will be evaluated. To extend the analytic models for including environmental features as well, another input than the velocity will be evaluated. One idea is to use the metabolic energy as proposed in [27] as the input workload. The metabolic energy formula allows to include the gradient, the subject's weight and road condition. Another study will investigate better learning parameters for the presented models. These learning approaches are quite sensitive to their learning configuration and their internal structure. It needs to be shown if the machine learning approaches can perform better by adjusting the learning parameters.

Acknowledgement. The authors gratefully acknowledge the on-going support of the Bonn-Aachen International Center for Information Technology. Furthermore, the authors would like to thank the subject for his support.

References

1. WHO: Demographic change, life expectancy and mortality trends in europe: fact sheet. In: The European Health Report 2012. World Health Organization (2012)
2. Nichols, M., Townsend, N., Luengo-Fernandez, R., Leal, J., Gray, A., Scarborough, P., Rayner, M.: European Cardiovascular Disease Statistics 2012. European Heart Network, Brussels, European Society of Cardiology, Sophia Antipolis (2012)
3. Graf, C., Bjarnason-Wehrens, B., Rost, R., Foitschik, T., Lagerström, D., Quilling, E.: Sport-und Bewegungstherapie bei inneren Krankheiten: Lehrbuch für Sportlehrer, Übungsleiter, Physiotherapeuten und Sportmediziner. Deutscher Ärzte-Verlag (2014)
4. Leveille, S.G., Guralnik, J.M., Ferrucci, L., Langlois, J.A.: Aging successfully until death in old age: opportunities for increasing active life expectancy. Am. J. Epidemiol. **149**(7), 654–664 (1999)
5. Baig, D., Javed, F., Savkin, A.: An adaptive h-infinity control design for exercise-independent human heart rate regulation system. In: 2011 9th IEEE International Conference on Control and Automation (ICCA) (2011)
6. Steffen, D., Bleser, G., Weber, M., Stricker, D., Fradet, L., Marin, F.: A personalized exercise trainer for elderly. In: 2011 5th International Conference on Pervasive Computing Technologies for Healthcare (PervasiveHealth), pp. 24–31 (2011)
7. Ludwig, M., Sundaram, A.M., Füller, M., Asteroth, A., Prassler, E.: On modeling the cardiovascular system and predicting the human heart rate under strain. In: Proceedings of the International Conference on Information and Communication Technologies for Ageing Well and e-Health (ICT4AgingWell) (2015)

8. Calvert, T., Banister, E.W., Savage, M.V., Bach, T.: A systems model of the effects of training on physical performance. IEEE Trans. Syst. Man Cybern. **SMC–6**, 94–102 (1976)
9. Hajek, M., Potucek, J., Brodan, V.: Mathematical model of heart rate regulation during exercise. Automatica **16**(2), 191–195 (1980)
10. Cheng, T.M., Savkin, A.V., Celler, B.G., Wang, L., Su, S.W.: A nonlinear dynamic model for heart rate response to treadmill walking exercise. In: 2007 IEEE International Conference on Engineering in Medicine and Biology Society (EMBS), pp. 2988–2991. IEEE (2007)
11. Cheng, T., Savkin, A., Celler, B.: Nonlinear modeling and control of human heart rate response during exercise with various work load intensities. IEEE Trans. Biomed. Eng. **55**(11), 2499–2508 (2008)
12. Paradiso, M., Pietrosanti, S., Scalzi, S., Tomei, P., Verrelli, C.: Experimental heart rate regulation in cycle-ergometer exercises. IEEE Trans. Biomed. Eng. **60**(1), 135–139 (2013)
13. Baig, D.Z., Su, H., Cheng, T.M., Savkin, A.V., Su, S.W., Celler, B.G.: Modeling of human heart rate response during walking, cycling and rowing. In: 2010 IEEE International Conference on Engineering in Medicine and Biology (EMBC), pp. 2553–2556. IEEE (2010)
14. Mohammad, S., Guerra, T.M., Grobois, J.M., Hecquet, B.: Heart rate control during cycling exercise using Takagi-Sugeno models. In: 18th IFAC World Congress. Milano (Italy) (2011)
15. Su, S., Wang, L., Celler, B., Savkin, A., Guo, Y.: Identification and control for heart rate regulation during treadmill exercise. IEEE Trans. Biomed. Eng. **54**(7), 1238–1246 (2007)
16. Koenig, A., Somaini, L., Pulfer, M.: Model-based heart rate prediction during Lokomat walking. In: Engineering in Medicine and Biology Society, EMBC 2009. Annual International Conference of the IEEE (2009)
17. Leitner, T., Kirchsteiger, H., Trogmann, H., del Re, L.: Model based control of human heart rate on a bicycle ergometer. In: Control Conference (ECC), 2014 European, pp. 1516–1521. IEEE (2014)
18. Corno, M., Giani, P., Tanelli, M., Savaresi, S.: Human-in-the-loop bicycle control via active heart rate regulation. IEEE Trans. Control Syst. Technol. **23**(3), 1029–1040 (2015)
19. Afonso, J.A., Rodrigues, F.J., Pedrosa, D., Afonso, J.L.: Automatic control of cycling effort using electric bicycles and mobile devices. In: Proceedings of the World Congress on Engineering 2015. IAENG (2015)
20. Velikic, G., Modayil, J., Thomsen, M., Bocko, M., Pentland, A.: Predicting the near-future impact of daily activities on heart rate for at-risk populations. In: 13th IEEE International Conference on e-Health Networking Applications and Services (Healthcom), pp. 94–97. IEEE (2011)
21. Sumida, M., Mizumoto, T., Yasumoto, K.: Estimating heart rate variation during walking with smartphone. In: Proceedings of the 2013 ACM International Joint Conference on Pervasive and Ubiquitous Computing, p. 245. ACM Press (2013)
22. Wang, L., Su, S.W., Celler, B.G.: Assessing the human cardiovascular response to moderate exercise: feature extraction by support vector regression. Physiol. Meas. **30**(3), 227 (2009)
23. Zhang, Y.: Monitoring, modeling, and regulation for indoor and outdoor exercises, Ph.D. thesis, University of Technology, Sydney (2013)

24. Yuchi, M., Jo, J.: Heart rate prediction based on physical activity using feedforwad neural network. In: International Conference on Convergence and Hybrid Information Technology, ICHIT 2008, pp. 344–350 (2008)

25. Xiao, F., Chen, Y., Yuchi, M., Ding, M., Jo, J.: Heart rate prediction model based on physical activities using evolutionary neural network. In: 2010 Fourth International Conference on Genetic and Evolutionary Computing, pp. 198–201. IEEE (2010)

26. Brzostowski, K., Drapala, J., Grzech, A., Swiatek, P.: Adaptive decision support system for automatic physical effort plan generation - data-driven approach. Cybern. Syst. **44**, 204–221 (2013)

27. Müller, F., Mülller, S., Helmer, A., Hein, A.: Evaluation of a generic heart rate model for exercise planning and execution across training modalities. In: Proceedings of the 7th German AAL Conference (2014)

28. Lefever, J., Berckmans, D., Aerts, J.M.: Time-variant modelling of heart rate responses to exercise intensity during road cycling. Eur. J. Sport Sci. **14**(1), S406–S412 (2014)

29. Busso, T., Denis, C., Bonnefoy, R., Geyssant, A., Lacour, J.R.: Modeling of adaptations to physical training by using a recursive least squares algorithm. J. Appl. Physiol. **82**(5), 1685–1693 (1997)

30. Hairer, E., Norsett, S., Wanner, G.: Solving Ordinary Differential Equations I. Nonstiff Problems. Springer Series in Computational Mathematics, 2nd edn. Springer, Berlin (1993)

31. Seal, H.L.: Studies in the history of probability and statistics. XV the historical development of the Gauss linear model. Biometrika **54**(1–2), 1–24 (1967)

32. Tabachnick, B.G., Fidell, L.S.: Using Multivariate Statistics, 5th edn. Allyn & Bacon, Inc., Needham Heights (2006)

33. Javed, F., Chan, G.S.H., Savkin, A.V., Middleton, P.M., Malouf, P., Steel, E., Mackie, J., Lovell, N.H.: RBF kernel based support vector regression to estimate the blood volume and heart rate responses during hemodialysis. In: International Conference of the IEEE Engineering in Medicine and Biology Society, pp. 4352–4355 (2009)

34. Van Der Malsburg, C.: Frank Rosenblatt: principles of neurodynamics: perceptrons and the theory of brain mechanisms. In: Palm, G., Aertsen, A. (eds.) Brain Theory, pp. 245–248. Springer, Berlin (1986)

35. Vapnik, V.: The Nature of Statistical Learning Theory. Springer, New York (1995)

36. Smola, A.J., Schölkopf, B.: A tutorial on support vector regression. Stat. Comput. **14**(3), 199–222 (2004)

Handling of Emergency Situations with Elderly Patients using Autonomous Mobile Robot and Smart Tablets

Syed Atif Mehdi[1]([⊠]), Shah Rukh Humayoun[2], Artem Avtandilov[1,2], and Karsten Berns[1]

[1] Robotics Research Lab, University of Kaiserslautern, Kaiserslautern, Germany
{mehdi,berns}@cs.uni-kl.de
http://agrosy.cs.uni-kl.de
[2] Computer Graphics and HCI Group, University of Kaiserslautern, Kaiserslautern, Germany
humayoun@cs.uni-kl.de, aavtandilov@gmail.com
http://hci.cs.uni-kl.de

Abstract. Knowing the up-to-date situation about the emergency environment and collaboration between the caregiver staff can be very useful in properly executing the rescue operations, especially in cases of elderly patients. The current advancements in the mobile autonomous robots and smart mobile devices (such as tablets) could provide better means to caregiver staff in handling these emergency situations more effectively and efficiently. In this paper, we present an overall solution to facilitate the caregiver staff to collaborate each other and interact with the elderly person in an emergency situation alone at home for properly executing the rescue operation. For this, we use a mobile app on smart tablet devices to make collaboration between the mobile Emergency Response Teams (ERTs) and the staff at central Health Service Center (HSC). Further, we provide communication mediums to facilitate the HSC and the ERTs to access and control over the robot in order to know the current situation of the emergency environment. We have performed a user evaluation study to check the usability of the developed mobile app. Results of the study indicate approximately the same accuracy and efficiency with users having no prior experience or training compared to experts users.

Keywords: Healthcare robotics · Interacting robots at home · Graphical user interfaces · Web-based interaction · Mobile platform · Evaluation study

1 Introduction

The elderly population in developed countries is steadily increasing [1]. In many situations these people live alone in their homes, which requires urgent assistance in case of some emergency situation that may happen to the person. Currently,

© Springer International Publishing Switzerland 2015
M. Helfert et al. (Eds.): ICT4AgeingWell 2015, CCIS 578, pp. 126–142, 2015.
DOI: 10.1007/978-3-319-27695-3_8

many research groups are devoting their efforts in developing personal robots that can perform several tasks in a typical home environment [2]. They focus normally on performing some activity in the home environment like fetching objects [3], folding laundry [4], etc. A few activities are also being performed in the range of tele-presence using robots [5–7]. These robotic platforms are connected to the Internet and can be used by authorized persons to investigate the health of an elderly person.

These robots can be more beneficial if they can provide support to the caregiver staff when an emergency happens to an elderly person. One such support would be to initiate the call to the caregiver staff informing about the situation, other possibilities would be to allow the robot to be remotely controlled without the need of any sophisticated hardware [8, 9]. Currently, only caregiver staff can remotely operate the robot and the Emergency Response Teams (ERTs) rely on the information provided to them.

However, the current smart mobile devices can play an important role in this regard. Targeting this concern, the main contribution of our work is development of a framework for establishing communication between the elderly person and the ERTs through the autonomous mobile robot and the smart tablets as well as enhancing the collaboration between the staff at central Health Service Center (HSC) and the ERTs. It is an extension to previously developed interfaces [9] where only staff at HSC was able to communicate with the elderly person using the mobile robot as a platform. We have performed evaluation studies of the developed mobile app at two stages: with the usability experts using the heuristic evaluation approach, and with users from different background in a controlled environment. Results of the user study depict that the users with no prior experience or training perform approximately the same as expert users.

The remainder of the paper is structured as follows: Sect. 2 provides an overview of the related work. The methodology of our solution for establishing communication between the caregivers and the emergency teams is described in Sect. 3. Section 4 provides the details about the mobile app that was developed to help the ERTs in collaborating with HSC and to access and control over the robot, ARTOS. Section 5 describes the communication between the different entities in the framework. Section 6 provides details of the conducted evaluation studies as well as discusses the results. Finally, Sect. 7 provides the conclusion and gives directions to the future work.

2   Related Work

Crucial parts of the emergency response environments are interaction between different entities in the environment and the channels available for this interaction. Many emergency services around the world have upgraded their hardware and software to meet the demand; however, vast majority of them still rely on the voice communication solutions as a primary source of information when most up-to-date information is required. Many previous works [10–12] have been tackling the issues in systematic approach to these frameworks.

Reddy et al. raised questions about the crisis management and how technologies could affect the emergency services [12]. They concluded that the teams of first responders and the service center have strong socio-technical aspect in interaction as well as pointing out that team-to-team and team-to-emergency sight communication are difficult to organize. On the other hand, Paul et al. found the role of technologies in the process as uncertain due to the opinion provided by the physicians participated in the study [11]. While Kyng et al. took a closer approach into how interactive such services could be, by setting specific challenges to the existing systems handling emergencies [10]. By illustrating the important role of the live video feed when handling an emergency, they provided sufficient proof that such solutions may be beneficial.

All the above-mentioned work took widely the theoretic approach to the problem; however, most of the work providing the real communication and engineering solutions are developed in the industry trying to meet market needs. Most pervasive approach in the industry developed by Motorola[1] provides a solution for the emergencies occurring in largely accessible public spaces, relies on the government's access to the CCTV recordings in real time, dedicated emergency channels and possibly a large impact. It aims at improving response times, enhancing safety for responders, and enabling better communication with emergency service center. This approach is based on a steady ground of communication technologies finely tuned for the needs of first responders; however, it lacks the individuality while tackling bigger problems. As much as it is effective in the aforementioned type of emergencies, it lacks individual approach when only one patient is endangered and does not provide interactive communication with the emergency scene.

Other solutions in the market like Mobile Solutions[2] and PK[3] take another approach trying to strengthen communication between different emergency services such as firefighters, medical personnel and law enforcement by providing extended database support with immediate access to records, dealing mostly with management problems. Mobility for the command center is showcased by PK. It can be installed on-site where it will serve as an authentication center and will issue tasks to all service members using hand-held devices.

As these industrial approaches target communication between the first responders and their command centers, they lack the channels that are difficult to organize [10], namely live video feed from the place where emergency occurred. These communication strategies consider facilitating interaction between the diseased person and the service center. Although this is important but they do not provide any framework for establishing communication between the emergency responding team and the person in distress, which could be helpful in better informing both the team and the person.

---

[1] http://www.motorolasolutions.com.

[2] http://www.elliottmobilesolutions.com.

[3] http://www.pk.nl.

3   Methodology

The main emphasis in this paper is to develop a framework for establishing communication channel between the Emergency Responding Team (ERT) and the elderly person in an emergency situation at the home environment. Since it is not known in advance which ERT will be able to reach the person at earliest; therefore, the emergency situation is reported to the Health Service Center (HSC). The HSC is then responsible to send the request to the ERTs and contact information is provided to only that ERT which accepts to undertake the responsibility. The responsible ERT can then communicate with the person using the autonomous mobile robot as a platform and navigate it in the home environment to understand the situation. Figure 1 gives an overview of the complete framework.

3.1   Autonomous Mobile Robot

The Autonomous Robot for Transport and Service (ARTOS) (see Fig. 2) has been developed at the Robotics Research Lab, University of Kaiserslautern in order to investigate challenges in providing services to elderly people living alone in their homes [13]. Due to its special design, the robot can easily navigate through narrow corridors and closely placed furniture in a typical household

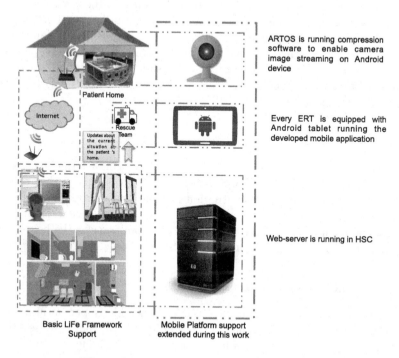

Fig. 1. Overview of the developed framework.

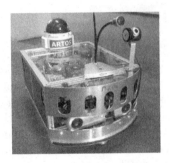

Fig. 2. Autonomous Robot for Transport and Service (ARTOS).

environment. It can be used to transport objects and establishing a communication link between the elderly person at home and remote caregivers using wireless Internet.

ARTOS is a differentially driven robot and capable of driving autonomously in the home environment. It generates an occupancy grid map of the environment using laser scanner and ultrasonic sensors [14]. The grid map is then used for path planning and navigating from one location to another. For accuracy in localization, RFID (Radio Frequency Identification) tags are installed under the carpet of the testing home environment and an RFID reader is placed under ARTOS to determine the current location of the robot in the environment [15]. The robot autonomously identifies key locations in the home environment to monitor the elderly person [16] and use this information to learn the daily routine of the person. The learned routine is then used for searching the person at different times of the day [17]. The robot can also be tele-operated by caregiver staff at HSC using a joystick in the Graphical User Interface (GUI) to observe the home environment [9].

3.2   Health Service Center

The Health Service Center (HSC) is the first point of contact that receives the emergency help request from ARTOS. After receiving the request, they can tele-operate the robot to evaluate the situation in hand and verify any false alarm. The GUI (see Fig. 3) at the center provides them with the view of the home using camera on the robot. After verification they can transfer the help request to the mobile teams to respond the emergency situation.

3.3   Emergency Response Teams

Emergency Response Teams (ERTs) respond to the elderly person in an emergency situation. After receiving the information from HSC, they can use ARTOS as a communication medium to evaluate the situation at home and to talk with the person in distress.

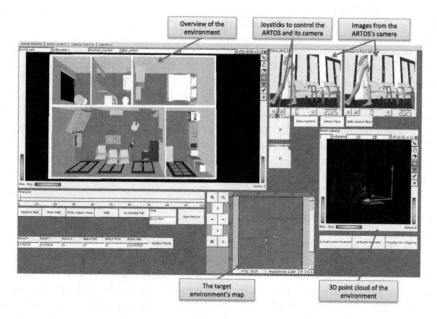

Fig. 3. The GUI at HSC that visualizes the elderly person's home environment and provides interactions to control ARTOS and the camera.

4   The Emergency Supporting Collaborative Mobile App

An Android application has been specifically developed, called **E**mergency **S**upporting **C**ollaborative **M**obile App (**ESCoM**), for the ERTs, to communicate with both HSC and ARTOS to receive most up-to-date information about the patient, their location, and the situation that they are about to get involved. Currently, this is an Android-based app and has been developed to target the smart tablet devices.

The functionality of the developed ESCoM app includes receiving live video image from ARTOS, joystick control of the robot to explore the environment, status reports to the HSC, database access for extended information about the patient, and navigation options.

The ESCoM app receives and interprets the messages received from the Google Cloud Messaging (GCM). The received message contains information about the patient, address and Skype id of ARTOS. ESCoM facilitates the ERT in determining the acceptance or rejection of the job. In case of acceptance, it further receives the information about the Skype id and IP address of the ARTOS. Once the vital information is received, ERT can directly communicate with the person in distress and does not require HSC, which significantly decreases the stressful job at HSC.

4.1   Emergency Request Handling

When a new request is generated by the HSC in order to notify all the available ERTs, the ESCoM app shows this notification to the ERT through its emergency request handling mode (see Fig. 4). This mode is intended to allow the ERT an opportunity to assess the situation as fast as possible in order to make a decision if they are capable to proceed with this emergency. All the basic functionalities (i.e., detailed information of the patient, navigation map to the patient home, an option to establish a Skype call with the patient, option to accept or decline the emergency request) can directly be accessed through this mode, and if needed, additional options can also be explored through the main menu.

4.2   Maps Navigation

ESCoM provides three map navigation options to the ERT in order to facilitate them in executing the rescue operation more efficiently and effectively. These three options are: the map for ARTOS location in the home environment, 3D map of the home environment, and the Google map to the elderly person home (see Fig. 5). These maps help the ERT to find the direction to the elderly person home as well as to find out the current situation of the home environment, which helps the ERT team to prepare for the rescue operation. Clicking any of them in the initial view in the ESCoM app, the corresponding map opens in the full screen mode. The Google map, which shows the direction to the elderly person home, is updated as the ERT moves towards the elderly person homes direction. The ARTOS location map is also updated as ARTOS moves around the home environment, which gives the ability to the ERT to monitor the home environment more effectively.

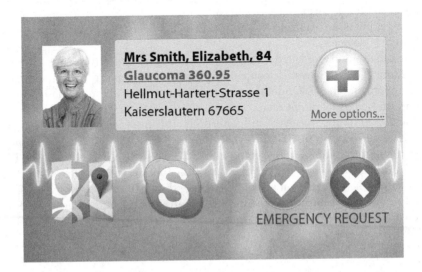

Fig. 4. ESCoM in the emergency request handling mode. It shows the different options available when the ERT gets an emergency handling request from HSC.

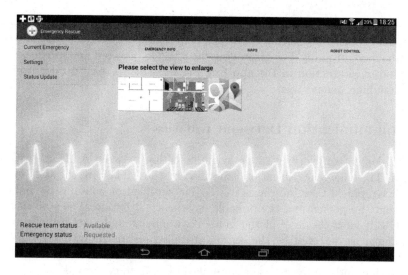

Fig. 5. Maps navigation mode in ESCoM app, which shows the availability of three maps, i.e.: map for ARTOS location in the home environment, 3D map of the home environment, and the Google map to the elderly person home.

4.3   Controlling ARTOS Camera and Navigation

ESCoM app also provides the facility to the ERT to view through the camera of ARTOS the current situation inside the elderly person home, as well as to control the movement of ARTOS in the environment. This is useful because it helps the ERT to know the live current situation of the home environment and

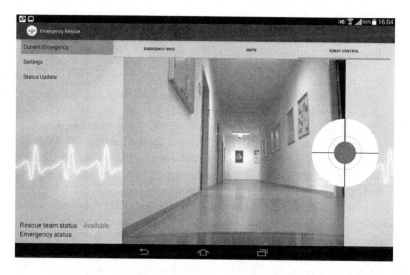

Fig. 6. The red joy-stick on the right-side of the screen is used to control the ARTOS movement, while the main view shows the current camera view of the ARTOS.

gives the facility to move the ARTOS in the area where they want to know the updated necessary information that could help them later in executing the rescue operation more properly. For controlling the ARTOS, ESCoM app provides a joy-stick kind of interaction in the app (see Fig. 6), which is easy to use from the tablet handling perspective.

5   Communication Between Entities

Figure 7 depicts an overview of the communication between ARTOS, HSC and ESCoM. The emergency situation is notified by the ARTOS to the staff at HSC on their Graphical User Interfaces (GUI). The notification contains the informa-tion about the person and the possible emergency situation. The staff member at HSC can view the map of the home environment and the obstacles in the environment as detected by the sensors installed on the robot using the GUI. The staff member can also remotely control the robot using the GUI to access the situation and rectify in case a false alarm has been generated.

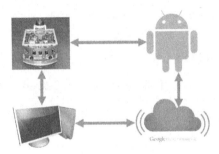

Fig. 7. Communication between the server at HSC and ESCoM using Google Cloud Messaging. Once information is received by the ESCoM app, the corresponding ERT can then directly communicate with ARTOS using the ESCoM app.

In case a valid emergency situation is recognized, the staff member at HSC can dispatch a message to notify all the ERTs or the nearest ERT about the situation. This is performed using the developed web server running at the HSC. The web server communicates with the Google Cloud Messaging (GCM) Services for dispatching the notification. The staff member can also monitor the location of each ERT by tracking their GPS coordinates in the integrated Google Maps. The web server at the HSC handles communication, feedback, status updates and database queries with the ESCoM app installed on the ERT tablet devices. It has been developed as a multi-user web interface that can automatically prioritizes lists of ERTs and pending emergencies, which allows HSC staff to act effectively and can decrease time needed to respond to an emergency request. Here we provide technical details of the communication channel between the ESCoM and ARTOS and between the HSC and ESCoM.

5.1   ESCoM-ARTOS Communication

The communication between the ARTOS robot and the ESCoM app is based on two communication modes: the third party application Skype Voice-over-IP call, and the direct publishing on ARTOSs ports for the camera image and to control the ARTOS movement (see Fig. 6).

The ESCoM app utilizes the IP and port addresses, which are fixed on both sides (i.e., on ARTOS side and on each of the ERTs tablet), for reading and sending the information. In the case of emergency request, the IP address of the specific ARTOS is passed over to all the ERTs or to specific ERTs. Further, access to the ports is granted immediately after the emergency request is sent to the ESCoM app in order to ensure best assessment of the situation. While the Joystick data on the ESCoM app (see Fig. 6) is transferred using the coordinates on the touch screen view to two ports relating to the X and Y coordinates of the current joystick touch. The camera image is encoded to JPG on ARTOS and published to the specific port, which is then decoded by ESCoM app into the image in order to live demonstrate in real time.

5.2   HSC-ESCoM Communication

The HSC is assumed to make all the decisions regarding allocation of a requested emergency to a specific ERT or a set of specific ERTs. In a normal circumstance, a set of available ERTs is suggested based on calculating their current positions to the emergency place. After allocation is complete, HSC broadcasts the emergency handling request through the Google Cloud Messaging (GCM) Service by matching the devices registration IDs at the corresponding ERTs. It is important to note that GCM contains only the devices registration IDs and passes the encrypted ID of the targeted ARTOS. ERTs are able to send an update directly to the HSC in order to know the current status of the emergency and the team. Again, these updates are sent through the secure network using the ERTs registration ID and the encrypted code of the targeted ARTOS.

6   The Evaluation Studies

The main contribution of our framework is establishing a communication platform between the health care staff at various levels (e.g., between the staff at HSC and the mobile response teams) and the elderly person at home. However, in our conducted evaluation studies we mainly focused on the ESCoM app that we have developed to be used by the mobile ERTs.

We conducted the evaluation studies at two stages. The first evaluation study was carried out with three usability experts using the heuristic evaluation [18, 19] approach. This evaluation ran on the first implemented prototype of the developed mobile app and the goal was to find out the possible usability flaws in the mobile app using the ten heuristics proposed by Nielsen [19]. Based on the results of this evaluation study by experts, we redesigned our mobile app user interface and made the suggested changes.

The second evaluation study was conducted with 10 participants having different background using the controlled task-based evaluation experiment approach. They were also given closed-ended and open-ended questionnaires at the end of experiment in order to know their feedback. These participants were mostly researchers and students from the University of Kaiserslautern, as the goal of the second evaluation study was to analyze whether the developed mobile app (which will be eventually used by ERTs) is easy to use without any prior training or expertise.

In the following subsections, we provide details of the conducted heuristic evaluation study followed by the user evaluation study in the controlled environment.

6.1   The Heuristic Evaluation Study

The heuristic evaluation study was done with three usability researchers from the Computer Graphics and HCI group of the University of Kaiserslautern. They evaluated the first implemented prototype of the ESCoM app using the ten heuristics and ranked the user interface giving a number from 0 to 4, where 0 means no problem at all while 4 means usability catastrophe [19]. The goal was to find out usability issues in the early stage of the ESCoM app development in order to improve the design and UI based on this evaluation.

A list of tasks were given to these experts consisted of the main features of the developed ESCoM app: i.e., managing settings, performing status updates, giving response to the emergency requests, establishing Skype call with the patient, sending feedback to the server, observing elderly person's household map, route planning with Google Maps, and controlling the ARTOS with joystick control option.

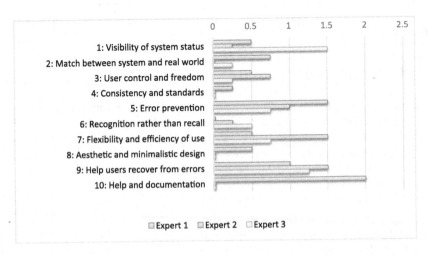

Fig. 8. The average score of the mobile app UI using the ten heuristics.

An introduction of the ESCoM app was given to these experts before they started to evaluate it. Further, the task description from the users' point of view was also given to them. They were also allowed to ask details about any UI element or task during the evaluation. In order to maintain the settings, the same person was given the chance to explain the ESCoM app and tasks during the evaluation. A form was given to these experts in order to record their feedback regarding the ten heuristics and their overall comments regarding any particular task or UI element.

Figure 8 shows the feedback of these three experts using the ten heuristics, where the score indicates the average of their given ranking in all tasks. The feedback indicated that some changes needed to be done for preventing errors and extending the visibility of the system status. However, there was not any major usability problem or usability catastrophe. The worst average grade of 2.0 from one expert was received in the category of help and documentation criteria. As the ESCoM app is intended to be used for professional purposes by ERTs, help and documentation must be sufficient for users with any level of competency and should provide in-depth review of the features. Other major issues were in the cases of fifth and ninth heuristics (average score of 1.25 and 1.08 by all experts, see Fig. 8), which indicated insignificant lack of clarity on how to prevent and recover from errors.

These experts also gave their suggestions for improving the usability of the ESCoM app, e.g., to introduce status fields of the rescue team and the current emergency. These suggestions were then analyzed and taken into account while developing the final version of the ESCoM app.

6.2   The User Evaluation Study

The goal of this conducted user evaluation study was to analyze whether the later version of the developed ESCoM app is easy to use without any prior training or expertise. Therefore, we were interested in finding out the effectiveness, efficiency, and user satisfaction aspects of our developed ESCoM app, as it will be used by ERTs for communicating with the HSC and the elderly person in the emergency situation. The following metrics were derived from the GQM model [20].

- *Metrics for Effectiveness:* We measure and compare the percentage of corrected completed tasks.
- *Metrics for Efficiency:* We measure and compare the time needed for completing each task.
- *Metrics for User Satisfaction:* We collect participants' feedbacks and compare them.

We combined these metrics as suggested by the Technology Acceptance Model [21]. For collecting the participants' feedbacks on how to improve the developed mobile app, we chose an open-ended questionnaire form in order to collect their comments. We formulated the set of hypotheses as:

- **H1:** We expect an effectiveness of more than 90 %, which means that in total participants accuracy of the completed task would be at least 90 %.
- **H2:** On average, both groups (i.e., the little or inexperienced group and the experienced group) achieve nearly the equal efficiency in completing the given tasks.
- **H3:** Participants agree that the developed mobile app is acceptable and useful for collaborating with HSC and ARTOS robot for handling the emergency request and for performing the rescue operation.

Study Design and Experiment Settings: Based on the identified goals and hypotheses, we designed this study as a controlled experiment under laboratory conditions with a maximum time frame of 45 min per participant. This allowed us enough time to have basic introduction explaining what is the idea behind the developed mobile app and what kind of environment participants will be interacting with.

We ran the study with 10 participants (6 males, 4 females), who were researchers and students from the University of Kaiserslautern having different backgrounds. Only one of them had prior experience in dealing with emergency situations. However, four of the participants had very little or no experience at all in using smartphones or smart tablets, while remaining six participants were experienced users of smartphones. Further, four of the participants never had any experience of robotics while five of them had some basic experience of robotics. The remaining one participant was an expert in robotics. The age range of participants in this study was from 20 to 44 years with a median of 27.8 years old.

The participants were given four tasks to complete one by one. Completion of the tasks was timed and participants had a chance to ask questions during the experiment in case they run into some technical difficulties or unable to complete the task by themselves. An evaluator was there to carefully write down the comments participants had given upon completion of each task in order to make sure that immediate feedback is possible. After tasks were completed, participants were presented with two questionnaires forms: closed-ended questionnaires form and open-ended questionnaires form. The closed-ended questionnaires form was based on nine questions, where each question offered a selection from six options on a Likert scale [22] (scale of 1 to 5 to show how much participants agree with the given statement and an additional option "Don't know"). The open-ended questionnaires form was aimed at general feedback in which the participants were asked to list any pros and cons they have identified in the developed mobile app and an opportunity to voice any other comments or suggestions.

The test was performed in the environment of the laboratory, with the participants seated in an office chair with no table and the tablet was freely in their hands. Participants were interacting with the ESCoM app using the standard touch features with no prior access to the platform in order to ensure no prior training or familiarity with the features.

Tasks Description: The test consisted of the following four tasks:

- **Task 1:** After an emergency request is issued: find the basic information about the patient, plan the route to the patient home on the Google map, and accept the emergency request.
- **Task 2:** After an emergency request is issued: initiate a Skype call and then decline the emergency request.
- **Task 3:** After accepting an emergency request: open additional options for the emergency situation, explore the map of the elderly patient household, control the ARTOS using the joystick, and navigate it to the patient.
- **Task 4:** As a team leader of the new started shift: enter your team details in the app settings and update the availability status.

Results and Discussions: In this subsection, we briefly discuss the results of the study. Overall, results of this conducted user evaluation study indicate satisfactory results in both groups.

From the effectiveness perspective, all of the participants were able to complete the tasks successfully and accurately, which shows a high rate of effectiveness and proves that the developed mobile app is easy to operate. This also proves our hypothesis H1 in which we were expecting that on average participants would be able to accurately complete the tasks or at least 90 % of the total tasks.

The results from the efficiency perspective (i.e., the time completion) are listed in Fig. 9, which shows the average time completion per task for the both groups (i.e., little or inexperienced users and experienced users). Participants from both groups do not show any significant differences in time completing any of the tasks. This demonstrates that the developed ESCoM app is easy to use and does not require much experience in order to complete the task. The main task (i.e., Task 3) that took most of the time was navigating the robot using the joystick and this is natural due to the speed of ARTOS. This brings us to the importance of the closed-ended questionnaires (see Table 1) and open-ended feedback from the participants. Even though most of the participants agreed that "It was easy to handle the robot with the joystick", the average grade of 3.8 is the lowest comparing to other features used in the developed mobile app. This was due to the security features of the robot navigation system and participants' unfamiliarity with the environment. In the real life scenarios, trouble of making yourself familiar with a new environment could facilitate emergency response team's actions when they arrive to the endangered person's house and when time matters the most. Overall, the results shown in Fig. 9 prove our hypothesis H2, in which we were expecting nearly the equal efficiency from the participants with little or no experience compared to the experienced participants.

When we look at the participants' feedback in the closed-ended questionnaires (see Table 1), we observe an average score of more than 4 in most of the cases, which shows high acceptance ratio of the ESCoM app amongst the participants. However, in question 3 (regarding the handling of robot through joystick) and question 4 (recovering from mistakes) we see a lower score. As described

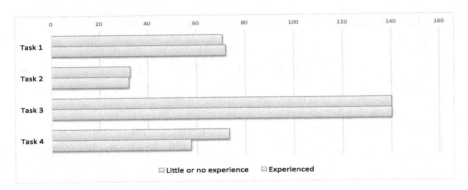

Fig. 9. Average time completion in seconds of participants in both groups.

Table 1. Participants' feedback in closed-ended questionnaires form. Here, 1 means "strongly disagree" and 5 means "strongly agree". The last column shows average score of all participants.

	1	2	3	4	5	N/A	Median
1: It was easy to see the current status of the system	0	1	1	5	3	0	4
2: It was easy to change Team availability status	0	1	2	0	7	0	4.3
3: It was easy to handle the robot with the joystick	0	2	2	4	2	0	3.8
4: It was easy to recover from mistakes	0	0	3	3	2	2	3.9
5: I found it easy to locate the needed features in the layout of the app	1	0	1	4	4	0	4
6: It was easy to complete provided tasks	0	1	0	3	6	0	4.4
7: It was clear from the icons the intended features they represent	0	0	1	2	7	0	4.6
8: I found the interface easy to use	0	0	1	6	3	0	4.2
9: I would recommend to use this system for emergency scenarios regularly	0	0	0	4	4	2	4.5

above, the first reason was in difficulty of handling the ARTOS while in the second case few of the participants were unfamiliar with the Android platform that allows users to go back to the previous stage through the Back navigation button. Overall, the results of participants in the closed-ended questionnaires also prove our hypothesis H3, in which we were expecting a high acceptance ratio from the participants.

Further, the feedback provided by the open-ended questionnaires reveals the particular features of the ESCoM app participants were or were not satisfied with. The open-ended questionnaires were built around the idea that the participant will give some basic feedback upon completion of every task and the evaluator will write it down, and after the participant completes all of the tasks he/she will be allowed to list pros and cons of the mobile app as well as giving any other general feedback. The collected open-ended feedback showed participants' appreciation towards the clarity in the GUI's visualization, namely the icons that were always reflecting the feature underneath it. They were also sharing their positive experience on how the interface was clear and reflecting the purpose of the ESCoM app. Among the cons participants were listing lack of the source for help when something was unclear and noting that they were ready to operate the ARTOS if it was moving around faster; therefore, saying that it was a little slower than they expected. One of the other common feedback responses was initial confusion with the log in mechanism for the team. Participants expected to be allowed to put their personal details in the mobile app, while they actually only needed to pick their identification (the badge number) to log in, which was specifically implemented to reduce time it takes to log in and avoid possible typos when entering the details.

7   Conclusions

This paper has demonstrated the use of a framework that can facilitate communication channel between an elderly person in emergency situation at a home environment, health service center and emergency responding teams. The autonomous mobile robot, AROTS, provides the channel for establishing this communication. The possibility of remotely controlling ARTOS to analyze the situation by moving the robot to different rooms and observe the images sent by the robot, enriches the user experience.

In the future, we plan to perform detailed evaluation studies in real environment settings to check the feasibility and effectiveness of the complete framework. Further, we also intend to develop a communication channel between different emergency responding teams in order to provide a better collaboration between these teams to tackle the emergency situation more effectively.

References

1. Lehr, U.: Population ageing. In: Online Handbook Demography. Berlin Institute for Population and Development (2007)
2. Wyrobek, K.: Towards a personal robotics development platform: rationale and design of an intrinsically safe personal robot. In: International Conference on Robotics and Automation, ICRA 2008 (2008)
3. Graf, B., Reiser, U., Hagele, M., Mauz, K., Klein, P.: Robotic home assistant Care-O-bot 3 - product vision and innovation platform. In: IEEE Workshop on Advanced Robotics and Its Social Impacts, Tokyo, pp. 139–144. IEEE (2009)
4. Ciocarlie, M., Hsiao, K., Jones, E.: Towards reliable grasping and manipulation in household environments. In: 12th International Symposium on Experimental Robotics, ISER (2010)
5. Kristoffersson, A., Coradeschi, S., Eklundh, K.S., Loutfi, A.: Sense of presence in a robotic telepresence domain. Univ. Access Hum.-Comput. Inter. **6766**, 479–487 (2011)
6. Merten, M., Bley, A., Schröter, C., Gross, H.M.: A mobile robot platform for socially assistive home-care applications. In: 7th German Conference on Robotics, ROBOTIK 2012, Munich, Germany, pp. 233–238 (2012)

7. Rumeau, P., Vigouroux, N., Boudet, B., Lepicard, G., Fazekas, G., Nourhachemi, F., Savoldelli, M.: Home deployment of a doubt removal telecare service for cognitively impaired elderly people: a field deployment. In: 3rd IEEE International Conference on Cognitive Infocommunications (CogInfoCom) (2012)
8. Deegan, P., Grupen, R., Hanson, A., Horrell, E., Ou, S., Riseman, E., Sen, S., Thibodeau, B., Williams, A., Xie, D.: Mobile manipulators for assisted living in residential settings. Auton. Robots Spec. Issue Socially Assistive Robot. **24**, 179–192 (2008)
9. Mehdi, S.A., Humayoun, S.R., Berns, K.: Life-support: an environment to get live feedback during emergency scenarios. In: Proceedings of the 8th Nordic Conference on Human-Computer Interaction: Fun, Fast, Foundational, Helsinki, Finland, pp. 935–938 (2014)
10. Kyng, M., Nielsen, E.T., Kristensen, M.: Challenges in designing interactive systems for emergency response. In: Proceedings of the 6th Conference on Designing Interactive Systems, DIS 2006, New York, NY, USA, pp. 301–310. ACM (2006)
11. Paul, S.A., Reddy, M., Abraham, J., DeFlitch, C.: The usefulness of information and communication technologies in crisis response. AMIA Annu. Symp. Proc. **2008**, 561–565 (2008)
12. Reddy, M.C., Paul, S.A., Abraham, J., McNeese, M., DeFlitch, C., Yen, J.: Challenges to effective crisis management: using information and communication technologies to coordinate emergency medical services and emergency department teams. Int. J. Med. Inf. **78**, 259–269 (2009)
13. Koch, J., Armbrust, C., Berns, K.: Small service robots for assisted living environments. In: VDI/VDE Fachtagung Robotik, Munich, Germany (2008)
14. Berns, K., Mehdi, S.A.: Use of an autonomous mobile robot for elderly care. In: Advanced Technologies for Enhancing Quality of Life, AT-EQUAL 2010, Iasi, Romania, pp. 121–126. IEEE Computer Society (2010)
15. Mehdi, S.A., Armbrust, C., Koch, J., Berns, K.: Methodology for robot mapping and navigation in assisted living environments. In: PETRA 2009: Proceedings of the 2nd International Conference on PErvasive Technologies Related to Assistive Environments, Corfu, Greece. ACM, New York (2009). ISBN-13: 978-1-60558-409-6
16. Mehdi, S.A., Berns, K.: Autonomous determination of locations for observing home environment using a mobile robot. In: 13th International Conference on Intelligent Autonomous Systems (IAS-13), Padua, Italy (2014)
17. Mehdi, S.A.: Using the human daily routine for optimizing search processes using a service robot in elderly care applications. Ph.D. thesis, Robotics Research Lab, Department of Computer Science, University of Kaiserslautern (2014)
18. Nielsen, J., Molich, R.: Heuristic evaluation of user interfaces. In: Proceedings Conference on Human Factors in Computing Systems, CHI 1990, Seattle, WA, USA, 1–5 April 1990, pp. 249–256 (1990)
19. Nielsen, J.: Enhancing the explanatory power of usability heuristics. In: Proceedings Conference on Human Factors in Computing Systems, CHI 1994, Boston, Massachusetts, USA, 24–28 April 1994, pp. 152–58 (1994)
20. Basili, V.R., Caldiera, G., Rombach, H.D.: The goal question metric approach. In: Encyclopedia of Software Engineering. Wiley (1994)
21. Venkatesh, V., Morris, M.G., Davis, G.B., Davis, F.D.: User acceptance of information technology: toward a unified view. MIS Q. **27**, 425–478 (2003)
22. Likert, R.: A technique for the measurement of attitudes. Arch. Psychol. **22**, 1–55 (1932)

Monitoring, Accessibility and User Interfaces

Home-Based Activity Monitoring of Elderly People Through a Hierarchical Approach

Xavier Rafael-Palou$^{(\boxtimes)}$, Carme Zambrana, Eloisa Vargiu, and Felip Miralles

eHealth Department, EURECAT, Barcelona, Spain
{xavier.rafael,eloisa.vargiu,felip.miralles}@eurecat.org,
carme.zambrana@ce.eurecat.org

Abstract. People that need assistance, as for instance elderly or disabled people, may be affected by a decline in daily functioning that usually involves the reduction and discontinuity in daily routines and a worsening in the overall quality of life. Thus, there is the need to intelligent systems able to monitor indoor and outdoor activities of users to detect emergencies, recognize activities, send notifications, and provide a summary of all the relevant information. To this end, several sensor-based telemonitoring and home support systems have been presented in the literature. Unfortunately, performance of those systems depends, among other characteristics, on the reliability of the adopted sensors. Although binary sensors are quite used in the literature and also in commercial solutions to identify user's activities, they are prone to noise and errors. In this chapter, we present a hierarchical approach, based on machine learning techniques, aimed at reducing errors from the sensors. The proposed approach is aimed at improving the classification accuracy in detecting if a user is at home, away, alone or with some visits. It has been integrated in a sensor-based telemonitoring and home support system. After being evaluated with a control user, the overall system has been installed in 8 elderly people's homes in Barcelona, results are presented in this chapter.

1 Introduction

Activity monitoring is an increasingly important research area due to the fact that it can be applied to many real-life, human-centric problems, such as eldercare and healthcare. Recent studies have shown that physical activities in daily life are an important predictor of risk of hospital readmission and mortality in patients with chronic diseases [1,2].

Monitoring users' activities allows therapists, caregivers, and relatives to become aware of user context by acquiring heterogeneous data coming from sensors and other sources. Moreover, activity monitoring provides elaborated and smart knowledge to clinicians, therapists, carers, families, and the patients themselves by inferring user habits and behaviour. Various methods of subjective and objective physical activity assessment tools have been developed. Subjective methods, such as diaries, questionnaires and surveys, are inexpensive tools.

© Springer International Publishing Switzerland 2015
M. Helfert et al. (Eds.): ICT4AgeingWell 2015, CCIS 578, pp. 145–161, 2015.
DOI: 10.1007/978-3-319-27695-3_9

However, these methods often depend on individual observation and subjective interpretation, which make the assessment results inconsistent [3]. On the other hand, objective techniques use remote monitoring techniques relying on sensors, such as home-automation, wearable and/or environmental ones [4].

A lot of telemonitoring systems have been proposed in the literature [5–7] and are currently adopted in real environments [8], enabling the healthcare provider to get feedback on monitored people and their health status parameters.

Sensor-based telemonitoring systems rely on a conjunction of sensors, each one devoted to monitor a specific status, a specific activity or activities related to a specific location. Sensor technology can range from vital signal devices – such as blood pressure monitors, heart rate monitors and devices which can measure body temperature – to sensors which can detect presence in a room or detect a door being opened [9]. Once all of the data have been recorded it is then necessary for data processing to take place to identify if the person requires a form of assistance since an unusual activity has been recognized. Of course, this requires a certain degree of intelligence which should take into consideration the current state of the environment, the performed activity and/or some physiological data [10]. Due to issues regarding personal privacy, technical installations, and costs of technology the most adopted sensors are anonymous binary sensors [9]. Binary sensors do not have the ability to directly identify people and can only present two possible values as outputs ("0" and "1"). Typical examples of binary sensors deployed within smart environments include pressure mats, door sensors, and movement detectors. A number of studies reporting the use of binary and related sensors have been undertaken for the purposes of activity recognition [11]. Nevertheless, sensor data can be considered to be highly dynamic and prone to noise and errors [12].

The increasing social demand for intelligent telemonitoring systems makes necessary to put more emphasis in activity recognition methods that deal with environments prone to errors [13]. In this chapter, we make a step forward in this direction by introducing a novelty and effective discriminative method based on machine learning. The goal is to discover the very initial but crucial information regarding the user location and recognition whether s/he is alone or with visits under complex, noisy and unstable environments. This chapter extends our previous work [14] presenting new experimental results regarding tests performed in 8 elderly people's homes in Barcelona.

The rest of the chapter, is organized as follows. In Sect. 2, we recall relevant work related to the partial detection of some of the activities that concern us and with settings similar to those presented in this work. Section 3 summarizes the adopted sensor-based telemonitoring and home support system, whereas Sect. 4 illustrates the adopted approach aimed at improving habit recognition. In Sect. 5, we first present comparisons among the proposed approaches to recognize if the user is alone or not, and, then, experimental results coming from elderly people's homes are shown. Section 6 ends the chapter with conclusions and future directions.

2 Related Work

There is a large literature on recognition of activities at home [15,16]. At the same time, we find a great variability in the settings of the experiments either in the number of sensors and their type, individuals involved or the duration thereof. Also noteworthy is the large amount of recognition techniques (supervised, either generative or discriminative; and unsupervised). This diversity makes it extremely difficult to compare performances and draw conclusive findings from those studies. Despite this high variability, it is noteworthy to mention that we have not found extensive studies that analyze altogether the detection of visits, presence or absence of users at home using wireless binary sensors. Even so; we report a number of different papers with different approaches related to the partial detection of some of the activities that concern us and with settings similar to those in our work.

A former study [11] already points out some of the difficulties in discriminating daily life activities based only on binary sensors activities. The automatic recognition system was based on rules defined from the context and the duration of the activities to identify. The data of the study were obtained from 14 days of monitoring activities at home. Although promising accuracy was achieved for some activities, detection tasks such as "leaving home" were nothing less than satisfactory with 0.2 of accuracy. This was because the activities were represented by rules directly defined on the firings outputted by single sensors (i.e. door switches); so they did not contemplate that could be activated for other reasons and in varying times, which made reduce their discriminating power.

A more exhaustive work regarding the use of switch and motion sensors for tracking people inside home is found in [17]. Tests were done with up to three simultaneous users. High performances were reported by the trained tracking models. However it is interesting to note that this type of sensors experimented occasional lag between "entering" a room and triggering a sensor; making to decrease the performance of the tracking models.

In [18] a more complex template learning model (SVM) was used to automatically recognize among 11 different home activities. The proposed technique was integrated in different sliding window strategies (e.g., weighting sensor events, dynamic window lengths, or two levels of window lengths). They used 6 months of data from 3 different homes in which activities such as "entering" or "leaving home" were monitored. From the best experimental settings the authors claimed accuracy for "entering" home about 0.80 of F1 but around 0.4 for "leaving" home tasks.

In a more extensive work [19], authors use Naïve Bayes (NB), Hidden Markov (HMM) models and Conditional Random Fields (CRF) for the activity recognition problem. In that study, 7 smart environments were used and 11 different data sets were obtained. Several activities were attempted to be recognized. Among others, we highlight "entering" and "leaving home" as relevant for our approach. Although they did not report specific accuracy for these activities, authors claimed an overall recognition performance on the combined dataset of 0.74 for the NB classifier, 0.75 for the HMM model, and 0.72 for the CRF using 3-fold cross validation over the set of annotated activities.

In [20], authors proposed a hybrid approach to recognize ADLs from home environments using a network of binary sensors. Among the different activities recognized "leaving" was one of them. The hybrid system proposed was composed by using an SVM to estimate the emission probabilities of an HMM. The results showed how the combination of discriminative and generative models is more accurate than either of the models on their own. Among the different schemes evaluated, the SVM/HMM hybrid approach obtains a significant 0.7 of F1, a notable better performance than the rest of approaches.

Detecting "multiple" people in single room by using binary sensors was already studied in an early work [21]. In that work, authors proposed a method based in Expectation Maximization Montecarlo algorithm. More recently [22], high accuracy (0.85) was reported on detecting visits at home using binary sensors. In that approach, authors used an HMM algorithm over the room events although not all rooms of the home were monitored.

3   The Sensor-Based Telemonitoring and Home Support System

To monitor users' activities, we developed a sensor-based telemonitoring and home support system (SB-TMHSS) able to monitor the evolution of the user's daily life activity. The implemented system is able to monitor indoor activities by relying on a set of home automation sensors and outdoor activities by using Moves[1]. Information gathered by the SB-TMHSS is also used to provide context-awareness by relying on ambient intelligence [23]. Monitoring users' activities through the SB-TMHSS gives us also the possibility to automatically assess quality of life of people [24,25]. In this Section, we briefly describe the SB-TMHSS, the interested reader may refer to [26] for further details.

The high-level architecture of the SB-TMHSS is depicted in Fig. 1. As shown, its main components are: home; healthcare center; middleware; and intelligent monitoring system.

At home, a set of sensors are installed. In particular, we use presence sensors (i.e., Everspring SP103), to identify the room where the user is located (one sensor for each monitored room); a door sensor (i.e., Vision ZD 2012), to detect when the user enters or exits the premises; electrical power meters and switches, to control leisure activities (e.g., television and pc); and pressure mats (i.e., bed and seat sensors) to measure the time spent in bed (wheelchair). The system is also composed of a network of environmental sensors that measures and monitors environmental variables like temperature, but also potentially dangerous events like gas leak, fire, CO escape and presence of intruders. All the adopted sensors are wireless z-wave[2]. They send the retrieved data to a collector (based on Raspberry pi[3]). The Raspberry pi collects all the retrieved data and securely redirects them to the cloud where they will be stored, processed,

---

[1] http://www.moves-app.com/.

[2] http://www.z-wave.com/.

[3] http://www.raspberrypi.org/.

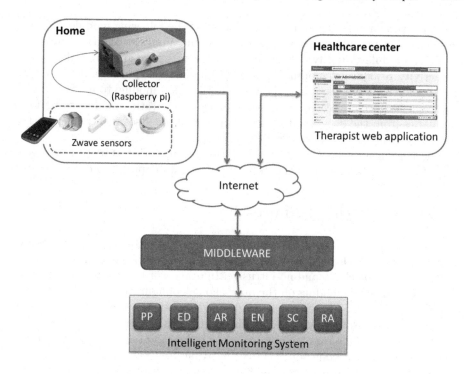

Fig. 1. Main components of the SB-TMHSS.

mined, and analyzed. The proposed solution relies on z-wave technology for its efficiency, portability, interoperability, and commercial availability. In fact, on the contrary of other wireless solutions (e.g., ZigBee), z-wave sensors are able to communicate with any z-wave device. Moreover, we adopt a solution based on Raspberry pi because it is easy-to-use, cheap, and scalable. We are also using the user's smartphone as a sensor by relying on Moves, an app for smartphones able to recognize physical activities and movements by transportation. Among the activity trackers currently on the market, we select Moves because it does not need user intervention being always active in background. The user interacts with the overall system through a suitable interface aware of end-user needs and preferences.

The middleware, which acts as a SaaS, is composed by a secure communication and authentication module; API module to enable the collector transmitting all the data from sensors to make them available to the intelligent monitoring system; and further utilities such as load balancing and concurrency.

In order to cope with the data necessities of the actors of the system (i.e., therapists, caregivers, relatives, and end-users themselves), an Intelligent Monitoring system has been designed. It is aimed to continuously analyzing and mining the data through 4-dimensions: detection of emergencies, activity recognition, event notifications, and summary extraction. In order to cope with these objectives, the Intelligent Monitoring system is composed of the following modules: PP, the pre-processing module to encode the data for the analysis; ED, the emergency detection module to notify, for instance, in case of smoke and gas leakage; AR, the activity recognition module to identify the location, position, activity- and sleeping-status of the user; EN, the event notification module to inform when a new event has been detected; SC, the summary computation module to perform summaries from the data and to provide quality of life assessment; and RA, the risk advisement module to notify risks at runtime.

The healthcare center receives notifications, summaries, statistics, and general information belonging to the users through a web application.

4   The Hierarchical Approach

The developed SB-TMHSS described above is aimed at recognizing activities and habits of a user who lives alone. One of the requirements of the implemented SB-TMHSS was to be cheap and no-intrusive. In other words, we use the minimum number of sensors depending on the user's home configuration, avoiding camera or wearable sensors. In particular, we decided to not use a camera for privacy reason and in accordance with the requirements coming from the end-user of the proposed system. Moreover, the sensors are wireless and rely on wi-fi connection to send data to the collector. Let us note that we decided to do not adopt a wired solution because is more expansive and intrusive. These requirements imply that we have to take into account with errors and noise coming from this configuration and to find a solution to avoid them. In fact, sensors are not 100 % reliable: sometimes they loose events or detect them several times. When sensors remain with a low battery charge they get worse. Moreover, also the Raspberry pi may loose some data or the connection with Internet and/or with the sensors. Also the Internet connection may stop working or loose data. Finally, without using a camera or wearable sensors we are not able to directly recognize if the user is alone or if s/he has some visits. Although, as said, a wireless solution is not 100 % reliable.

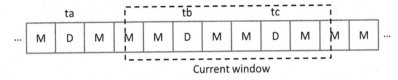

Fig. 2. An example of the sliding window approach, where M means "motion event" and D means "door event".

In order to solve this kind of limitations with the final goal of improving the overall performance of the SB-TMHSS, we propose an approach based on machine learning techniques. In this initial solution, we only consider motion and door sensors. The intelligent monitoring system continuously and concurrently listens for new data in a given window, according to a sliding window

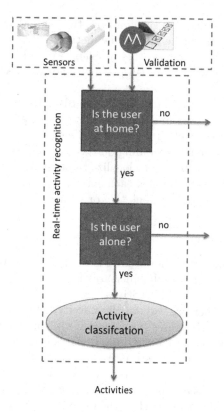

Fig. 3. The hierarchical approach in the activity recognition module.

approach [27]. For each window, data are pre-processed and analyzed. As an example, let us consider the Fig. 2 where once the current window recognizes a door event at time tb, it looks for the previous one in the window or before (in the example ta). Then, the period from that door events (i.e., $tb-ta$) is classified by the hierarchical classifier. Seemly, when the event tc has been recognized, the period from tb and tc is classified. Finally, the period from tc to the end of the window is classified. In case of no door events have been recognized, the period from ta to the end of the window is classified.

The hierarchical approach, depicted in Fig. 3, is composed of two levels. The upper is aimed at recognizing if the user is at home or not, whereas the lower is aimed at recognizing if the user is really alone or if s/he received some visits.

4.1 Is the User at Home?

The goal of the classifier at the upper level is to improve performance of the door sensor. In fact, it may happen that the sensor registers a status change (from closed to open) even if the door has not been opened. This implies that the SB-TMHSS may register that the user is away and, in the meanwhile, activities are detected at user's home. On the contrary, the SB-TMHSS may register that the user is at home and, in the meanwhile, activities are not detected at user's home. To solve, or at least reduce, this problem, we built a supervised classifier able to recognize if the door sensor is working well or erroneous events have been detected.

First, we revised the data gathered by the SB-TMHSS searching for anomalies, i.e.: (1) the user is away and at home some events are detected and (2) the user is at home and no events are detected. Then, we validated those data by relying on Moves, installed and running on the user smartphone. In fact, Moves, among other functionality, is able to localize the user. Hence, using Moves as an "oracle" we build a dataset in which each entry is labeled depending on the fact that the door sensor was right (label "1") or wrong (label "0").

4.2   Is the User Alone?

The goal of the classifier at the lower level is to identify whether the user is alone or not. The input data of this classifier are those that has been filtered by the upper level, being recognized as positives.

To build this classifier, we rely on the novelty detection approach [28] used when data has few positive cases (i.e., anomalies) compared with the negatives (i.e., regular cases); in case of skewed data. In particular, we rely on the approach presented in [29] that tries to estimate a function f that is positive on the dataset and negative on the complement. The functional form of f is given by a kernel expansion in terms of a potentially small subset of the training data; it is regularized by controlling the length of the weight vector in an associated feature space. The expansion coefficients are found by solving a quadratic programming problem, which we do by carrying out sequential optimization over pairs of input patterns.

5   Experimental Results

Before installing and testing the overall SB-TMHSS to recognize activities of elderly people, we evaluated the system in 1 able-bodied 40 years-old woman's home in Barcelona ("Control User", shortly CU). To train and test the proposed approach, we consider a window of 4 months for training and evaluation (training dataset) and a window of 1 month for the test (testing dataset). Experiments have been performed at each level of the hierarchy. First, we performed experiments to identify the best supervised classifier to be used at the upper level of the hierarchy. Subsequently, we applied the novelty detection algorithm on the data filtered by the classifier at the upper level, to validate the classifier at the lower one. Finally, we measure the performance of the overall approach.

Once evaluated the overall hierarchical solution, under the umbrella of a collaboration with the CVI[4], we installed the TMHSS in 8 elderly people's homes for evaluation and testing from a total of 41 days.

---

[4] http://www.cvi-bcn.org/en/.

Table 1. Results for the high-level classifier during the training (T) and evaluation (E) phase.

Classifier	Parameter (s)	Accuracy (T)	Accuracy (E)
LR	$C = 0.005$	0.945 ± 0.09	0.885
SVM	$\gamma = 0.01, C = 1.0$	0.945 ± 0.09	0.885
SVM	$\gamma = 1.0, C = 0.452$	0.853 ± 0.12	0.943
SVM	$\gamma = 0.05, C = 0.452$	0.930 ± 0.11	0.885
SVM	$\gamma = 0.01, C = 0.257$	0.945 ± 0.09	0.885
RF	$n\_estimators = 5$	0.943 ± 0.09	0.942
RF	$max\_features = 12$	0.930 ± 0.09	0.942
AB	$n\_estimators = 15$	0.918 ± 0.10	0.823

5.1   Experimental Results with the Control User

Is the User at Home? First of all, we build the training dataset with door events (gathered by the door sensor) in a window of 4 months. Those data have been then validated by relying on the information coming from Moves. The entries are manually labeled in two classes *Correct data* and *User not at home* according to the following criteria:

– *Correct data:* 0 if the data gathered from the door sensor differs from the data gathered from Moves; 1 otherwise.
– *User not at home:* 0 if the user is at home; 1 otherwise.

First, we define and implement a rule-based system to verify if an approach based on rules may help in improving the overall performance. The results coming from the rule-based system have been then compared with those manually validated using Moves. Unfortunately, results show a very few improvement with an accuracy of 77 %. Thus, we decide to implement a supervised classifier.

The data labeled as 1 for the class *Correct data* have been used to extract the following features:

– number of motion events divided by their duration, calculate after a door event (from $t = i$ door event to $t = i + 1$ door event) [Feature 1];
– number of motion events divided by their duration, calculated before a door event (from $t = i - 1$ door event to $t = i$ door event) [Feature 2];
– number of motion events happened during minute before a door event ($t = i$) [Feature 3];
– number of motion events happened during the 2 min before a door event ($t = i$) [Feature 4];
– number of motion events happened during the 5 min before a door event ($t = i$) [Feature 5];
– number of motion events happened during minute after a door event ($t = i+1$) [Feature 6];

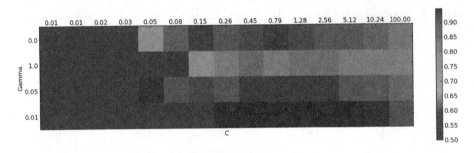

Fig. 4. Cross-validation results of the different setting of parameters in the SVM classifier.

- number of motion events happened during the 2 min after a door event ($t = i + 1$) [Feature 7];
- number of motion events happened during the 5 min after a door event ($t = i + 1$) [Feature 8].

The dataset is then used to train four well-representative and successful families of supervised classifiers [30]: a Logistic Regression (LR) classifier, a Support Vector Machine (SVM), a Random-Forest (RF) and an AdaBoost (AB).

The dataset has been divided in a training and in an evaluation set and a 10-fold cross-validation method has been used. The classifiers have been then tested with an independent dataset. Table 1 shows results during the training phase and evaluation phase. As shown, the best performance has been obtained by relying on the SVM (with $\gamma = 1.0$ and $C = 0.452$), see Fig. 4, which shows different combination of the parameters kernel coefficient (γ) and penalty parameter of the error term (C).

The best classifier has been then used with the testing dataset and, on average, it obtained a F_1 of 0.97 and an accuracy of 0.968. Finally, it showed an improvement of 20 % with respect to the rule-based approach.

Is the User Alone? The data filtered by the classifier at the upper level, belonging to the monitored window of 4 months, are the training dataset of the classifier at the lower level. The corresponding dataset is composed by 57 normal instances (i.e., the user was alone) and 8 anomalies (i.e., the user received visits).

First of all, also in this case, we defined and implemented a rule-based classifier to verify if a rule-based approach could solve this problem. The adopted rules together with the number of anomalies detected by each one are the following:

- Number of movement events every 60 s greater than 6: 23 anomalies detected;
- Number of movement events every 60 s greater than 10: 1 anomaly detected;
- Simultaneous movement events: 20 anomalies detected;
- Simultaneous movement events in less 2 s: 23 anomalies detected;
- Maximum number of movement events in 60 s greater than 6 or simultaneous moves in less 2 s: 28 anomalies detected;

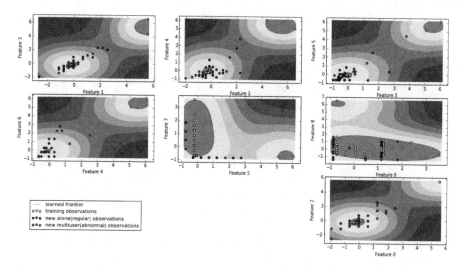

Fig. 5. Feature analysis of select novelty outlier method.

Table 2. Results for the classifier at the lower level. The table reports the classification error calculated as the ratio between the number of detected anomalies and the number of instances in the dataset.

Parameter (s)	Error (T)
$\nu = 0.01, \gamma = 0.1$	0.0701
$\nu = 0.01, \gamma = 0.5$	0.0877
$\nu = 0.01, \gamma = 1$	0.1578
$\nu = 0.05, \gamma = 0.1$	0.0877
$\nu = 0.05, \gamma = 0.5$	0.0877
$\nu = 0.05, \gamma = 1$	0.1403
$\nu = 0.1, \gamma = 0.1$	0.1052
$\nu = 0.1, \gamma = 0.5$	0.1052
$\nu = 0.1, \gamma = 1$	0.1403
$\nu = 0.5, \gamma = 0.1$	0.4912
$\nu = 0.5, \gamma = 0.5$	0.5087
$\nu = 0.5, \gamma = 1$	0.4912

- Maximum number of movement events in 60 s greater than 6 or simultaneous moves: 21 anomalies detected.

Since the rule-based approach is not able to correctly recognized anomalies, we use, also in this case, an SVM classifier (one-class SVM with RBF, non linear). The following features have been considered:

- maximum number of motion events in intervals of 60 s [Feature 1];

Table 3. Results of the overall hierarchical approach with respect to the rule-based one.

Metric	Rule-based	Hierarchical	Improv.
Accuracy	0.80	0.95	15 %
Precision	0.68	0.94	26 %
Recall	0.71	0.91	20 %
F_1	0.69	0.92	23 %

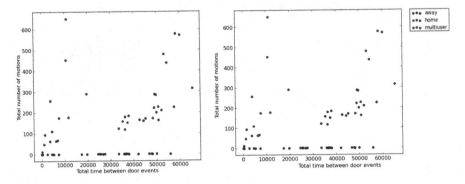

Fig. 6. Comparison between real labeled data and data classified by the hierarchical approach.

- maximum number of motion events in intervals of 120 s [Feature 2];
- maximum number of motion events in intervals of 180 s [Feature 3];
- number of motion events happened in a range of 5 s [Feature 4];
- number of motion events happened in a range of 2 s [Feature 5];
- number of motion events happened simultaneously [Feature 6];
- minimum number of seconds between two consecutive motion events [Feature 7];
- average of seconds between two consecutive motion events [Feature 8].

The classifier has been trained by considering the normal instances and then evaluated introducing the anomalies. Figure 5 shows the results obtained considering two features at time. In particular, for each pair of features the frontier, the training observations and the observations in case of normal instances (regular) or anomalies (abnormal) have been shown. Table 2 shows the overall results.

Results during the evaluation phase show that the system is able to correctly recognize all the anomalies. According to the obtained results, we select the classifier with the regularization parameter $(\nu) = 0.01$ and $\gamma = 0.1$.

Similarly to the classifier at the upper level, the system has been tested with the data coming from the 1-month window of monitored events. Results showed an average accuracy of 0.94.

Table 4. Experimental results from the installation at CVI.

Metric	Is the user at home?	Is the user alone?
Accuracy	0.95	0.68
Precision	0.98	0.64
Recall	0.98	0.74
F_1	0.98	0.68

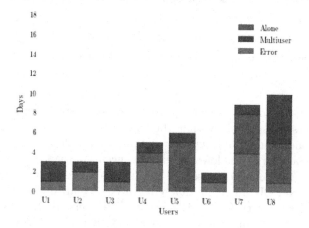

Fig. 7. Results of the classifier at the lower level for each monitored user (U1 - U8).

Overall Results. Once both classifiers have been trained, we tested the performance of the overall approach with the testing dataset corresponding to a window of 1 month. We compared the overall results with those obtained by using the rule-based approach in both levels of the hierarchy. Results are shown in Table 3 and point out that the proposed approach outperforms the rule-based one with a significant improvement.

To highlight the performance of the proposed approach, let us consider the Fig. 6 that shows a comparison between the real data, labeled during the validation phase (on the left), and the data classified by relying to the approach proposed in this paper (on the right).

5.2   Experimental Results with Elderly People

The overall SB-TMHSS has been installed in 8 elderly people' homes (7 women) over 65 years old, thanks to the collaboration of CVI, a centre aimed at assisting dependent elderly and/or people with disabilities using supporting products and technology to improve the quality of life and facilitate autonomy and security in the home. To test the hierarchical classifier, we asked all the users to daily answer to two questions: "how many times do you go out home today?" and "how many visits do you receive today?". Results are showed in Table 4, moreover,

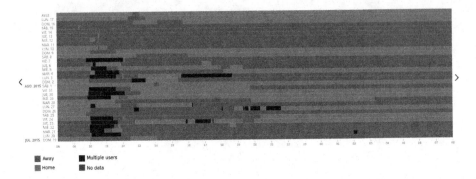

Fig. 8. Example of results in recognizing if U8 is at home or away or if she received some visits.

Fig. 7 shows the performance of the classifier at the lower level for each of the monitored users. Results show that the classifier at the upper level has very good performance, comparable with those calculated with data from CU. On the contrary, the classifier at the lower level is less accurate than the system working with CU data. This can be caused by multiple factors. For instance, habits of elderly people and CU might be different. In particular, during the monitored period, CU received very few visits whereas CVI users received visits more or less daily (e.g., the cleaning lady). Moreover, elderly people might have different activity patterns at home from younger people, e.g., normally they move slowly and tend to have long inactivity periods. Also, home and room configuration might affect to the classifier performance, i.e., short distances between rooms generates more measurements than in broad places.

Finally, as an example of how the data are transmitted to the caregivers for activity monitoring, Fig. 8 summarizes a month of activity of U8.

6   Conclusions and Future Directions

Community based living, often alone with intermittent care, creates possible scenarios of risks for all individuals. When cognitive changes are likely to have taken place it is crucial to understand what the risks may be and monitor these. To monitor users at home, we develop a sensor-based system which is able to gather data and report on the stability and evolution of the user's daily life activity. Unfortunately, performance of sensor-based telemonitoring and home support systems depends, among other issues, on the reliability of the adopted sensors. It is particularly true in the case of a wireless and binary sensors are adopted. To solve this problem, we presented a hierarchical approach, based on machine learning techniques, aimed at improving the recognition of the presence of the user at home and, being interested in monitoring people that live alone, if the user is alone or received some visits. Results with the Control User clearly show an high discriminative performance improvement of 15 % with respect to a rule-based solution.

To test the approach in the field, the system has been installed in 8 elderly people's homes in Barcelona. Results confirm the effectiveness of the system, especially on detecting home user presence and its absence, and, at the same time, highlight the need of some improvements in order to reach the same results obtained with the Control User. In particular, we envisage three main directions that may be gone through: (i) to train the system with more data and to use a different approach for the classifier at the lower level, as for instance an ensemble of novelty detection algorithms; (ii) to train the system with data from elderly people instead of selecting a younger woman, as Control User; and (iii) to personalize the classifier for each user, i.e., to have a different system for each user, trained with data coming from the user her/himself. Finally, we are considering to test the approach also with people with acquired brain injury.

Acknowledgements. The research leading to these results has received funding from the European Community's, Seventh Framework Programme FP7/2007-2013, Back-Home project grant agreement n. 288566.

References

1. Yohannes, A.M., Baldwin, R.C., Connolly, M.: Mortality predictors in disabling chronic obstructive pulmonary disease in old age. Age Ageing **31**, 137–140 (2002)
2. Pitta, F., Troosters, T., Spruit, M.A., Decramer, M., Gosselink, R.: Activity monitoring for assessment of physical activities in daily life in patients with chronic obstructive pulmonary disease. Arch. Phys. Med. Rehabil. **86**, 1979–1985 (2005)
3. Meijer, G.A., Westerterp, K.R., Verhoeven, F.M., Koper, H.B., ten Hoor, F.: Methods to assess physical activity with special reference to motion sensors and accelerometers. IEEE Trans. Biomed. Eng. **38**, 221–229 (1991)
4. Warren, S.: Wearable and wireless: distributed, sensor-based telemonitoring systems for state of health. Can. J. Anim. Sci. **80**, 381–392 (2000)
5. Carneiro, D., Costa, R., Novais, P., Machado, J., Neves, J.: Simulating and monitoring ambient assisted living. In: Proceedings of ESM (2008)
6. Corchado, J., Bajo, J., Tapia, D., Abraham, A.: Using heterogeneous wireless sensor networks in a telemonitoring system for healthcare. IEEE Trans. Inf. Technol. Biomed. **14**, 234–240 (2010)
7. Mitchell, M., Meyers, C., Wang, A., Tyson, G.: Contextprovider: context awareness for medical monitoring applications. In: Conference Proceedings of the IEEE Engineering in Medicine and Biology Society (2011)
8. Scanaill, C.N., Carew, S., Barralon, P., Noury, N., Lyons, D., Lyons, G.M.: A review of approaches to mobility telemonitoring of the elderly in their living environment. Ann. Biomed. Eng. **34**, 547–563 (2006)
9. Nugent, C.D., Hong, X., Hallberg, J., Finlay, D., Synnes, K.: Assessing the impact of individual sensor reliability within smart living environments. In: IEEE International Conference on Automation Science and Engineering, CASE 2008, pp. 685–690. IEEE (2008)
10. Cook, D.J., Das, S.K.: How smart are our environments? An updated look at the state of the art. Pervasive Mob. Comput. **3**, 53–73 (2007)

11. Tapia, E.M., Intille, S.S., Larson, K.: Activity recognition in the home using simple and ubiquitous sensors. In: Ferscha, A., Mattern, F. (eds.) PERVASIVE 2004. LNCS, vol. 3001, pp. 158–175. Springer, Heidelberg (2004)
12. Ranganathan, A., Al-Muhtadi, J., Campbell, R.H.: Reasoning about uncertain contexts in pervasive computing environments. IEEE Pervasive Comput. **3**, 62–70 (2004)
13. Jafari, R., Encarnacao, A., Zahoory, A., Dabiri, F., Noshadi, H., Sarrafzadeh, M.: Wireless sensor networks for health monitoring. In: The Second Annual International Conference on Mobile and Ubiquitous Systems: Networking and Services, MobiQuitous 2005, pp. 479–481. IEEE (2005)
14. Rafael-Palou, X., Vargiu, E., Serra, G., Miralles, F.: Improving activity monitoring through a hierarchical approach. In: The International Conference on Information and Communication Technologies for Ageing Well and e-Health (ICT 4 Ageing Well) (2015)
15. Van Kasteren, T., Noulas, A., Englebienne, G., Kröse, B.: Accurate activity recognition in a home setting. In: Proceedings of the 10th international conference on Ubiquitous computing, pp. 1–9. ACM (2008)
16. Ye, J., Dobson, S., McKeever, S.: Situation identification techniques in pervasive computing: a review. Pervasive Mob. Comput. **8**, 36–66 (2012)
17. Wilson, D.H., Atkeson, C.: Simultaneous tracking and activity recognition (STAR) using many anonymous, binary sensors. In: Gellersen, H.-W., Want, R., Schmidt, A. (eds.) PERVASIVE 2005. LNCS, vol. 3468, pp. 62–79. Springer, Heidelberg (2005)
18. Krishnan, N.C., Cook, D.J.: Activity recognition on streaming sensor data. Pervasive Mob. Comput. **10**, 138–154 (2014)
19. Cook, D.J.: Learning setting-generalized activity models for smart spaces. IEEE Intell. Syst. **27**(1), 32–38 (2010)
20. Ordónez, F.J., de Toledo, P., Sanchis, A.: Activity recognition using hybrid generative/discriminative models on home environments using binary sensors. Sensors **13**, 5460–5477 (2013)
21. Wilson, D., Atkeson, C.: Automatic health monitoring using anonymous, binary sensors. In: CHI Workshop on Keeping Elders Connected, Citeseer, pp. 1719–1720 (2004)
22. Nait Aicha, A., Englebienne, G., Kröse, B.: How lonely is your grandma?: detecting the visits to assisted living elderly from wireless sensor network data. In: Proceedings of the 2013 ACM Conference on Pervasive and Ubiquitous Computing Adjunct Publication, pp. 1285–1294. ACM (2013)
23. Casals, E., Cordero, J.A., Dauwalder, S., Fernández, J.M., Solà, M., Vargiu, E., Miralles, F.: Ambient intelligence by atml: rules in backhome. In: Lai, C., Giuliani, A., Semeraro, G. (eds.) Emerging Ideas on Information Filtering and Retrieval, DART 2013: Revised and Invited Papers (2014)
24. Vargiu, E., Fernández, J.M., Miralles, F.: Context-aware based quality of life telemonitoring. In: Lai, C., Giuliani, A., Semeraro, G. (eds.) Distributed Systems and Applications of Information Filtering and Retrieval, DART 2012: Revised and Invited Papers. Springer, Heidelberg (2014)
25. Vargiu, E., Rafael-Palou, X., Miralles, F.: Experimenting quality of life telemonitoring in a real scenario. Artif. Intell. Res. **4**, 136–142 (2015)
26. Rafael-Palou, X., Vargiu, E., Dauwalder, S., Miralles, F.: Monitoring and supporting people that need assistance: the backhome experience. In: Lai, C., Giuliani, A., Semeraro, G. (eds.) DART 2014: Revised and Invited Papers (2014, in press)

27. Datar, M., Gionis, A., Indyk, P., Motwani, R.: Maintaining stream statistics over sliding windows. SIAM J. Comput. **31**, 1794–1813 (2002)
28. Markou, M., Singh, S.: Novelty detection: a review? Part 1: statistical approaches. Sig. Process. **83**, 2481–2497 (2003)
29. Schölkopf, B., Platt, J.C., Shawe-Taylor, J., Smola, A.J., Williamson, R.C.: Estimating the support of a high-dimensional distribution. Neural Comput. **13**, 1443–1471 (2001)
30. Fernández-Delgado, M., Cernadas, E., Barro, S., Amorim, D.: Do we need hundreds of classifiers to solve real world classification problems? J. Mach. Learn. Res. **15**, 3133–3181 (2014)

HCI for Ageing Populations

Mapping Memories for People with Dementia

Alina Huldtgren[1,2](✉), Anja Vormann[2], and Christian Geiger[2]

[1] Eindhoven University of Technology, Eindhoven, The Netherlands
a.huldtgren@tue.nl
http://alina.huldtgren.com
[2] University of Applied Sciences Duesseldorf, Duesseldorf, Germany

Abstract. Due to the demographic change and the world's ageing populations the number of people with dementia will rise dramatically in the coming years. Dementia impacts all areas of daily life and, in particular, memory and communication. Although technology provides promising means to address these challenges, few technologies have been successfully developed that empower the people with dementia instead of simply leaving them in a passive position. We aim specifically to design interactive systems that can be used by people with dementia, e.g., as part of reminiscence therapy to remember the past and communicate with others. In this paper, we present our research and design approach and exemplify the design case of the interactive Reminiscence Map. This is a tangble interface developed in collaboration with a person with early stage dementia. We present results and further developments based on field research and focus groups with care experts.

Keywords: Tangible interaction · Multimedia · Reminiscence therapy

1 Introduction

Demographic changes and longer life expectancy lead to a growing number of people with dementia. In 2014, about 36 million people worldwide had Alzheimers or a related form of dementia, the highest percentage living in Western Europe (www.alzheimers.net/resources/alzheimers-statistics/). Over the course of the disease, dementia severely impacts memory, speech and language, thinking, orientation and social behaviour. As a result people with dementia have difficulties in all areas of daily life, often become frustrated and experience lower life quality. In extreme cases such frustrations can even lead to challenging behaviours such as unrest, aggression or apathy [3]. Unfortunately, there are no medical treatments available at this point to cure the disease. Instead psychosocial interventions play an important role in order to increase the wellbeing of people with dementia. Psychosocial interventions include among others reminiscence, reality orientation or memory training, which have proven to positively and sustainably influence challenging behaviours of people with dementia [4].

Technology has recently started to play an important role in the area of care, mostly in the form of assistive systems for the home care context (AAL). Systems for people with dementia often put users in a passive role, e.g., when GPS

© Springer International Publishing Switzerland 2015
M. Helfert et al. (Eds.): ICT4AgeingWell 2015, CCIS 578, pp. 165–184, 2015.
DOI: 10.1007/978-3-319-27695-3_10

is used to track lost people [12]. However, "[l]iving with dementia presents a range of challenges ripe for creative applications of technology" [2]. We believe, that the currently prevailing technology-led developments miss some important values and needs of people with dementia. Design approaches involving the target group resulting in technical artefacts for people with dementia have a higher potential to address these people's needs. Especially in the area of designing for reminiscence, maintaining personhood and communication new media technologies can be utilized in supportive ways.

In the so-called NutzerWelten (English: UserWorlds, www.nutzerwelten.de) project our interdisciplinary team investigates ways in which multimedia technologies can be utilized to support and enhance the experience of reminiscence and communication for people with dementia. Until now, we conducted exploratory field research in different settings (e.g. a care home, day care and support groups) and developed a number of interactive multimedia artefacts to be deployed in these settings for observation and discussion with people with dementia and caregivers. We intend to identify design possibilities for multimedia technologies that integrate smoothly into people's daily lives.

In this paper we focus, in particular, on one design case that emerged from our field research in a local care home. We describe the development of a tangible interface called Reminiscence Map - a physical map allowing the user to select a timespan and remember places and stories from that time. The map was co-developed with a person with early-stage dementia as a personalized artefact and discussed in an interview with the person, a focus group with the caregivers in the institution and workshop with practitioners and experts in dementia care, technology and other disciplines. Especially the first focus group led to further developments, e.g. adding a digital interface allowing the caregivers to find overlap in the places and stories of care home residents.

Similar to Wallace et al., our Reminiscence Map acts "[a]s a tool of enquiry it revealed valuable spaces for design in dementia that have wider implications for interaction design" [17]. In particular, the analysis of the case surfaced themes for technology design (e.g., leaving a legacy) that had not originally been considered.

2   Background

In the following we frame our design case with the recent insights from literature that informed this research. In particular, we will first describe types of psychosocial interventions, and in specific reminiscence, for people with dementia. Next, we will outline the state-of-the-art of technologies for reminiscence, in specific the role of tangible computing.

2.1   Psychosocial Interventions for People with Dementia

Researchers investigating dementia, especially those following a person-centred perspective [9], believe that the symptoms [e.g. depression and fears] and behaviours [e.g. unrest, aggression, wandering] of demented individuals are not solely a manifestation of the underlying disease process, but also reflect the social and environmental context, as well as the demented individuals perceptions and reactions. Psychosocial interventions can address these factors [8]. Psychosocial interventions are even more important in light of the limited success of pharmaceutical interventions for dementia. Kasl-Godley and Gatz [8] reviewed the six main psychosocial interventions for people with dementia: psychodynamic approaches, reminiscence and life review therapy, support groups, reality orientation, memory training and cognitive/behavioural approaches. Each intervention targets particular factors and addresses different goals. For instance, while psychodynamic approaches are helpful for gaining insight in the intra-psychic experiences of the individual, reminiscence and life review help with creating interpersonal connections. Behavioural approaches as well as memory training, on the other hand, are less concerned with the subjective experiences, but target specific cognitive deficits. Generally, it is recommended to involve others in these interventions in order to increase social contact, interpersonal communication and psychological health [8].

2.2 Reminiscence Therapy

As dementia progresses individuals experience memory loss, disorientation and in later stages a loss of their sense of self. As such, it becomes increasingly difficult for them to engage in meaningful activities, although this is of high importance for their quality of life [20]. It is argued that reminiscence may be particularly important for demented individuals psychological health given that the progressive deteriorating nature of the disease erodes the ability to achieve present successes and makes individuals increasingly dependent on past accomplishments for a sense of competency [8]. Since remote memory is usually spared for large parts of the dementia process, people are often able to recall events from the past. Furthermore, abilities like sensory awareness (response to stimuli like visual, audio and tactile), musical responsiveness and emotional memory (ability to experience rich emotions) are thought to persist in dementia, making reminiscence through audio-visual and tactile media possible. Even while processing memories may be compromised due to the brain damage, reminiscence can still provide structure in developing relationships or engaging with others [21].

2.3 Technologies and Reminiscence Therapy

Although contrary to our findings in field research, where caregivers used mainly non-technical objects such as images (e.g. photographs or photo books) and objects from the past (e.g. old packaging of products), as well as sensory stimulation through smells and haptics (e.g. different materials) or music, a recent literature review [10] on technologies used in reminiscence therapy points to many research projects in which ICT was used, e.g. in the form of displaying media on touch screens or projections. The purposes of using technology in reminiscence, as analyzed by Lazar et al. are two-fold: either to account for deficits such as motoric problems or memory loss or to harness strengths, such as emotional memory. In the CIRCA project [5] researchers created a multimedia application using video, photo and music to support one-to-one reminiscence sessions. The interface was meant to be used by caregivers initiating conversations with people with dementia. The authors reported positive results from user testing. More recent work of the same research team [1] focused on multimedia for leisure. For instance, computer-generated 3D environments provided means for people with dementia to enjoy environments they once liked, but cannot visit anymore, e.g. a garden or a pub. Similarly, [15] utilized immersive 3D technology, in particular Unity3D and the Kinect, to create environments for reminiscence and meaningful activities (like gardening). However, people with progressed dementia had problems with the interaction. Lazar and colleagues [10] found that "Challenges include that many of the systems described in the study require technical expertise for setup or operation and may not be ready for independent use." We would like to address this specifically in our project by designing tangible everyday objects that hide the technology in a way that users do not need any technical expertise and even people with dementia can interact with them.

2.4   Tangible Computing and Reminiscence

Although it has already been recognized [19] that tangible computing is a way to approach a person-centered model (for designing technology for seniors), the exploration of tangible computing within the area of reminiscence is so far limited to a handful of examples that we briefly outline.

One of the early works on using tangible interfaces designed specifically for older adults to trigger reminiscence was Nostalgia [13], which consisted of an old radio and an interactive textile runner with a diamond pattern. The runner was augmented with hidden switches that could be pressed to select music and news from different timespans ranging from 1930 to 1980. A preliminary evaluation showed that people at the care home were able to interact with the device and that it triggered discussions about the old news and singing along with the music. Another medium, familiar to seniors, that was deemed suitable for broadcasting information for reminiscence to people in a care home was the television. For instance, Waller and colleagues [19] designed an extended television that extended the regular TV program with specific care home internal and personal programs. The TVs were installed in the rooms of the residents as well as the communal rooms to allow for private reflection as well as communication between residents about the programs, which showed among others, old TV series, pictures from the care home and events, and personal photographs. In the unstructured evaluations, the authors found some proof that people used the TVs and also discussed the contents. However, especially people with dementia had problems using the standard remote controls. For one such person a tangible remote in form of a photo frame was built. This could be used by the person, but was rarely approached by herself (without a caregiver).

More recent work targeted specifically to people with dementia was done by Wallace and colleagues [17,18]. In the Tales of I project [17] they designed a system comprised of a wall cabinet holding several snow globes that encased objects relating to topics like soccer, holidays or local and a television cabinet with a mold to hold a globe. Through RFID chips in the globe the TV could read the correct topic and start the related film. Films were created from footage ranging back to the 1930s. In addition, personal content for each client could be played via a USB stick. In this project authors found that in the hospital setting where the system was installed in a common living room, it provided a sense of home for clients and visiting relatives, which was often lacking in the sterile hospital rooms. Through a sense of home and familiarity anxiety and challenging behaviors could be reduced. In addition, staff members were able to see a client more as a full person, when that person reconnected to a sense of self through the films.

In the Personhood project [18], in-depth research into the lived experiences of people with dementia was done through designing design probes with and for a couple, in which the wife suffered from dementia. Based on this research interactive jewelry was designed for reminiscence and providing a sense of self, through old media (like personal photographs in a locket) and personalized tangible artifacts (like a brooch made of old dresses).

3   Project Context

In the NutzerWelten project, researchers and designers from four disciplines (Media Technologies, Design, Electrical Engineering and Social Sciences) collaborate on solutions for people with dementia. Our research focuses on empowering people with dementia, on the one hand, through active integration in the design processes of new care technologies, and, on the other, by designing solutions adapted to their abilities, needs, and values.

While from the perspective of informal caregivers providing safety is one of the most important functionalities of technology [16], experiences from studies with people with dementia emphasized other values. For instance, communication with their surrounding, having a meaningful activity and establishing a connection with biographic aspects were identified to be of highest relevance for a good quality of life [2,14,20]. Therefore, we focus on the design of technical aids to improve communication of people with dementia and people in their surrounding, preferably through the use of biographic aspects.

3.1   Research and Design Approach

Designing for and with people with dementia is a sensitive endeavour and requires an empathic design approach [11]. Emphasizing and creating trust is a first crucial step. This is why we had a 3-months period in the beginning of the research process (Fig. 1) in which we gathered information about dementia through literature research, expert presentations and documentary films about dementia to sensitize the design team. Before visiting the field to get a first hand perspective we engaged in an activity where all design team members reflected about how

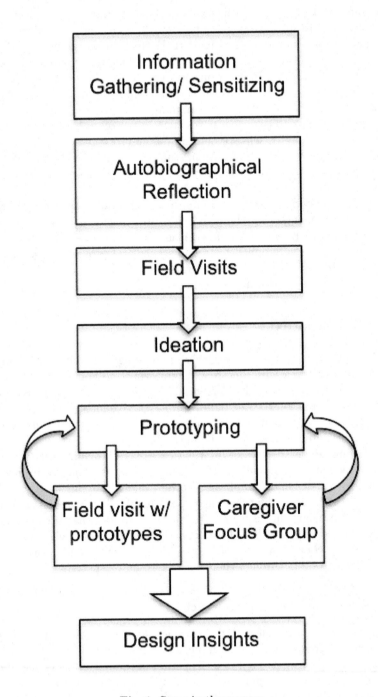

Fig. 1. Steps in the process.

they reminisce, which objects trigger memories and in what ways. First field visits were organized in close collaboration with the dementia service network in our city. We established contacts to several welfare organizations and were transferred to the key personnel in care homes (with stationary and day care) and in support groups for people with dementia. Several of our team members did (participant) observations and conducted either semi-structured interviews with caregivers or relatives or narrative interviews with people with dementia in order to elicit insights into their lived world.

In particular, these first visits were done during the course of one month and included: one visit of a day care centre with observation and an interview with a care manager, three visits to a care home including observations and interviews with five residents, several visits to three different support groups including participant observations (i.e. our team members took part in the group's program), two interviews with relatives of people with dementia in their homes, one visit to a geronto-psychiatric unit of a care home with observations as well as one interview with a caregiver and one with a resident, and, last, one interview of a person suffering from Lewy-body dementia. Observations focused mainly on the (everyday) activities people engaged in, and on the interactions between people. The interviews with caregivers focused mainly on the practical aspects of care, the communication and ways to support people in reminiscence. Interviews with relatives were similar, but focused also on the emotional aspects of dealing with the disease of their loved ones, from diagnosis and throughout the course of dementia. Interviews with people with dementia in the care homes focused on biographical aspects and life experiences.

The collected data in form of video, photos, field notes and interview transcripts were discussed with the team and used in the ideation phase, where two brainstorming sessions were held involving around 6–7 groups of ca. three people each time (mixed groups composed of students and researchers with backgrounds in design, HCI, computer sciences and media technologies). The result was a large number of ideas ranging from interactive furniture (mirrors, carpets), technology-enhanced everyday objects (stuffed animals, books) to completely newly designed artefacts. While some ideas focused more on functional aspects such as day planning, we selected a final set of ideas based on their expected potential to foster reminiscence and communication, their expected ease of use for people with dementia, their practicality to deploy in different environments and their potential to stimulate different senses.

All selected ideas contained multimedia content (video, audio, light and sound), either as original content from the past, recorded stories about the past, or recorded content from today that reminded of events or places of personal significance (e.g. videos of favourite places). Six prototypes were built in the next phase that were subsequently tested with people with dementia in the field. We also conducted a focus group with two caregivers and two care managers in the care home, where we presented all prototypes and discussed ideas for further development. Each prototype was assigned to a different caregiver in the home, who helped with the further development and provided test settings with residents. After an iteration of improving the prototypes, we presented them in an expert workshop with 20 participants comprising caregivers, dementia support group leaders, professionals from dementia research, social workers, and technology researchers. In the 1.5-hour workshop participants first experienced all six probes in an interactive exhibition and then discussed different aspects of the prototypes in focus groups of 5 people each.

Results of this process on all six objects will be published elsewhere. In the following, we will focus on discussing one of the designs in detail to show how this interactive object gave us insights into the needs of a person with dementia and possible uses of interactive technologies in the care home. These perspectives are valuable for interaction design in this domain.

4   Design Case: Interactive Reminiscence Map

4.1   Design Concept

In one of the interviews in the first field research phase, a person suffering from mild dementia (called Mrs Smith in this paper) expressed the wish to own a world map to mark all places that she had visited to use it as a memory aid for later.

A map is a well-known visual representation of geography. While physical maps provided guidance to people in the past, people use digital maps today. In addition, a map is a good interface for memory support as combining location information with visual images [or in our case recorded stories] might allow people to better situate past activities in context [7]. In the brainstorming session the idea was developed to create an interactive map for Mrs Smith to not only support memories of places, but also have a way to situate Mrs Smith's stories in

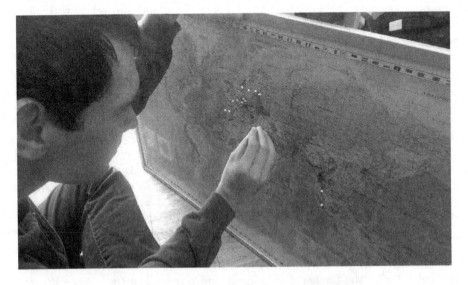

Fig. 2. Marking places on map during interview.

time and place. While this could easily be built as, e.g., a tablet app, we decided to use a physical map, in order to create an intuitive user interface that does not require another digital device. A common representation for time is a time bar. To set a certain time span of a persons life, we therefore, used a horizontal time slider with a big handle. To indicate visited cities in the chosen time span we used LEDs placed on the map.

The stories told by Mrs Smith in the first interview were audio-recorded and could be played back for the chosen time span by pressing a physical button with a speaker icon. During the interview analysis we found that some important temporal information was missing to place all narratives onto the timeline. Therefore, a second interview was conducted to focus on the stories and missing dates and to reconstruct all events in Mrs Smiths life. Some difficulties occurred in this process due to memory deficits, but with the help of a world map and small needles (Fig. 2) most narratives could be placed in time.

4.2 Prototype Implementation

The prototype was developed as a tangible interface. The basis is a printed map of 60 × 40cm that was glued onto a corkboard (Fig. 3). The size was chosen as a balance between providing a good resolution and portability. The lightweight material allowed the map to be easily held with one hand.

The heart of the technical backend (Fig. 4) is an Arduino Uno microcontroller equipped with an audio-shield. All places were marked on the map using coloured

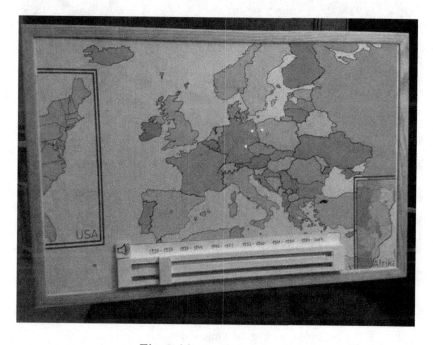

Fig. 3. Map prototype front.

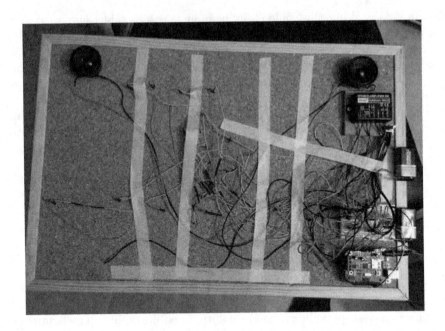

Fig. 4. Map prototype back.

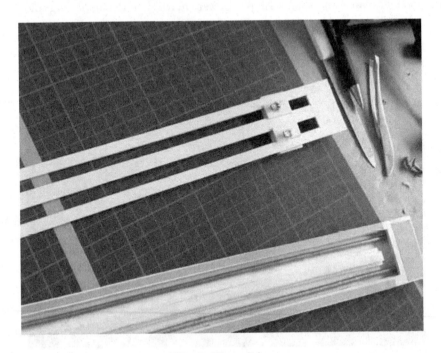

Fig. 5. Time slider.

3 mm LEDs to be controlled through the time slider, which was build from 6 mm cardboard (Fig. 5), a material used in advanced prototyping. We used two parallel rods on the backside of the slider, one made from copper and a plastic one wrapped with resistance wire (10). The current of 5 V sent through the wire drops depending on the position of the handle, which makes the electricity flow back through the copper rod that is connected to the analogue input of the Arduino. When a new position is retrieved, the respective LEDs are controlled via the PWM output of the Arduino (using a shift register to control several LEDs in parallel). The speaker button is implemented as a simple push button with a cardboard interface. For each time span an audio file is saved on the micro SD card inside the audio- shield. When the speaker button is pushed, the position of the time slider is used to access the particular audio file. We used two miniature speakers (1 W) hidden on the backside of the map for audio output.

4.3 Mrs Smith's Life

At the time of the interview Mrs Smith was 94 years old. She was born in 1920 in Landsberg an der Warthe, Germany, which belongs to Poland nowadays (and is called Gorzw Wielkopolski). At the age of six she moved to Berlin where she had a carefree childhood. Early on she found her calling in taking care of children and already worked for a year in a Kindergarten when she was 13. Later on, she became a paediatric nurse and worked for the Red Cross during World War II. After the war, she felt the desire to see the world. Working as a nanny for rich people this could be satisfied. Her first appointment as a nanny for a jeweller's children brought her to Italy and Switzerland, the second to the US and Denmark, and a third to Germany and France. In her stories today she refers to the children she took care of as her children. During her retirement she continued traveling including trips to Russia, Scandinavia, Spain, Singapore and Africa. Today Mrs Smith lives in the care home where she is mainly tied to her bed due to limited mobility. She suffers from mild dementia, which was hard to recognize for us in the first conversations, but became apparent due to the difficulties when placing her stories in time.

4.4 Feedback from Field Visits

Feedback from Mrs Smith. We visited Mrs Smith a third time after the prototypical interactive map was built. We did not intend to do a controlled user test, but to elicit her feedback in an unstructured interview. The following vignette (based on the first authors field notes) presents what happened.

We enter Mrs. Smiths room together with a caregiver. We greet Mrs. Smith and she immediately recognizes my colleague. I introduce myself and take a seat. Mrs. Smith asks curiously if there was already something to see. My colleague brought her a map as a gift to keep, where he marked all her visited cities. Mrs. Smith is surprised to find all the places on it. "Even Breslau is on it!" Then she says proudly, "but I was also in Africa." It seems that she had not immediately seen that Africa was also on the map. My colleague points it out to her and Mrs Smith starts telling a story about her stay in Africa.

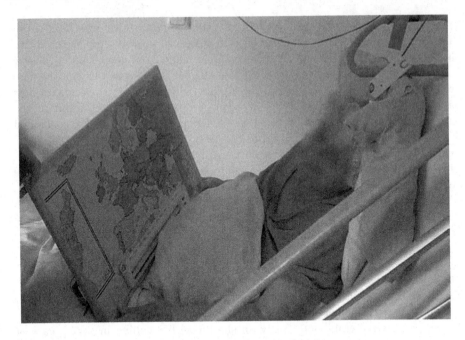

Fig. 6. User test with Mrs Smith.

After her story is told my colleague demonstrates the interactive prototype and shows how it works by setting the slider on 1920. An LED lights up. "That's when I was born! Mrs. Smith exclaims. After the demonstration Mrs. Smith teases the caregiver in the room "That's great! Do you also have a map like this?" He says jokingly that there would not be any lamps lighting up on a map for him, because he has not seen much of the world.

"What are you going to do with the map? Will it be in an exhibition?" Mrs. Smith asks. My colleague is surprised and says that our intention was to improve the map and maybe give it to her, but Mrs Smith likes her idea of making the map and her stories publicly available. "It could be interesting to other people to hear my stories," she says. Later in the conversation Mrs. Smith suggests that we could also give the map to her GP, who seems to be dear to her, after she passed away. "Then he can remember my stories." she says her eyes filling with tears.

The conversation stops, it is quiet. Mrs. Smith looks at the marked places on the map and suddenly begins a new story about when she was crossing the border between the GDR and West Germany and was held captive at the border. A bit later, we hear another story about Mrs. Smith crossing the Atlantic Ocean by boat, to which we listen reverently.

When my colleague invites her to try out the map herself she takes it in her hand (Fig. 6). With shaky fingers she moves the slider and places it on a timespan. She presses the speaker button to start the audio, but the sound is a little low, so that she has to move the map closer. When we ask her whether it is strange to hear her own voice telling the stories, she says that she does not care. The caregiver suggests that we take a photo together. When he lifts her bed, she starts fiddling with her t-shirt to get ready for the picture.

Throughout our visit Mrs. Smith looks at the map several times and starts telling different stories about the places marked on the map. In another conversation break, I take the initiative to learn something about Mrs. Smith. I see on the map that she has also visited Scandinavia, where I once lived. I ask her about a place there, and she tells us an exciting story about a bus trip through Scandinavia.

In many of her stories she mentions 'her children', but when I ask her about how many children she had, she says surprised "None! I took care of children of rich people." She reflects for a while and continues, "Others had families and I travelled around a lot. That's life. I made the best of mine." In this moment she looks content.

After 30 min had passed since we arrived, she seems tired and we politely say our goodbyes and tell her that we will improve the map further and show her the results again, if we may. She smiles and says "Of course, if I can be of help. You are always welcome."

We will return to different aspects from this field visit in the discussion section.

Feedback from Experts in Care and Technology. Besides discussing the map with the target user we also conducted workshops with caregivers and other experts. A focus group with four caregiver managers was held in the care home where Mrs Smith resides. In a two-hour session we first explained the goals of our research and then showcased all interactive prototypes, among these the Interactive Reminiscence Map. Each object led to discussions about its multimedia contents, the user interface and possible uses in different contexts in the care home.

In addition, we ran a workshop with 20 experts comprising caregivers, dementia support group leaders, professionals from dementia research, social workers, and technology researchers. In the 1.5-hour workshop participants first experienced all six prototypes in an interactive exhibition and then discussed different aspects of the prototypes in focus groups of 5 people each. Criticism, comments and ideas were written on post-it notes which were collected for later analysis. Focus group sessions were also audio-recorded.

The complete results on all six prototypes will be published elsewhere. Instead we focus here on the feedback that we received for the Reminiscence Map. Two aspects about the map were highlighted in the discussions: (1) its potential as a communication trigger via places, in particular, also for group sessions and (2) its appearance (virtual/physical).

Although the map was originally designed as a person-tailored object for Mrs Smith, her comment about sharing her story with others, led to a reflection that the map could be developed further in a way that could make several residents' life stories accessible to other stakeholders and in other contexts, including, for instance, other residents, visitors, family members and caregivers in the home or even outside the context of the home in museums or online. To handle several residents the idea for a digital version (see next section) was developed. Especially the caregivers were fond of this idea since a digital version could contain extended functionality to highlight places where several people have once been, thereby providing cues for communications in groups of people with dementia.

"That sounds good, because it is often like that. I often visit places and then I usually find a conversation partner, one person was also in Austria, the other knows Mallorca, the other Southern Germany. It is great [to communicate] via the cities." (female caregiver). Another aspect is that people may have visited the same places, but at different times, which would allow for conversations about how places changed over time. "I think this is great, because it connects people. There is this outsider status that people with dementia still have that would be released a bit, because there are places where everyone has once been. Places, everyone has memories about. Even if some loose their memories slowly, there are still points that connect people. I think this is a great image." (female care manager).

Adding functionality to the map, such as finding overlap between users or showing additional media content (e.g. photos from the times people visited places) would be easier in a digital system using a screen instead of a physical map. While the caregivers were not entirely against this idea, it was mentioned that the old physical maps (that were used in geography classes in school) would also be useful, as residents would still remember them. Such old maps could serve as an inspiration, one caregiver said, even if the interface was digital. Also the option of a combination of a digital system for several residents and personalized physical representations for single residents to keep was discussed. This way two different stakeholder groups would be catered for.

During the expert workshop several advantages of a digital system were highlighted, such as the possibility to add multimedia material such as photographs or videos to the places to allow for more vivid memories. In addition, a virtual map could also show changing country borders over time, thereby allowing people with dementia to relate better to the places as they were in the past, and younger generations to learn about a country's history. Concerns of the experts about the digital system were mainly centered around collecting the data (in form of stories, photographs, etc.) and making it available through the system. Caregivers, on the other hand, were less concerned as the collection of data about residents could go hand in hand with biographical work done in most care homes.

5   Digital Prototype

Based on the feedback from caregivers to implement a version of the Reminiscence Map that can provide additional functionality suited for triggering group communication we implemented a first simple, but fully functional digital system (running in a web browser). The life stories of several people with dementia, called narrators, can be stored in this system in form of a list of life events relating to a time and place. On the upper part of the screen a worldmap and a time slider can be found, in the lower part one or more narrators can be selected and a list of their events is displayed (see Fig. 7). The system allows a user to enter new narrators, new events for a narrator as well as delete events or narrators. When a narrator and a time span is selected the associated events are updated and the world map shows the location of the events in the form of colored circles (one color per narrator). By selecting several narrators it is possible to see on the map if two or more people visited the same place during the same time. To find out if people visited the same place, but at different times, the event list can be used. Clicking on a person or an event opens up an additional dialog giving more details about the person or the event including images and audio.

This prototype was tested in small scale usability test with six participants aged 27 years on average, who were asked to follow three scenarios (adding a narrator, deleting an event for any narrator, adding an event for the created narrator). All participants were able to finish the tasks without further instruction and participants rated the system positively. The prototype was displayed alongside the tangible map in the expert workshop described above to retrieve feedback on the idea of two different interfaces for the Reminiscence Map.

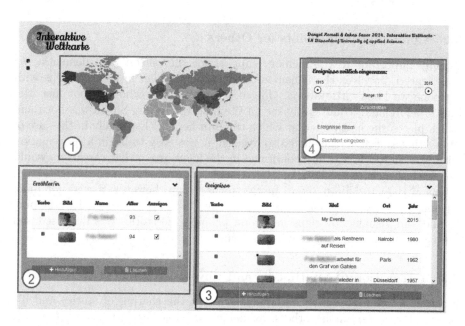

Fig. 7. Digital prototype for caregivers. (1) Map panel. (2) Narrator panel. (3) Event panel. (4) Time panel.

6   Discussion

In the following we present the themes that emerged from the field research, and, in particular, the feedback we received from Mrs Smith, the caregivers and experts on the Reminiscence Map.

6.1   Trigger of Memories

In the session with Mrs Smith we noticed that even the non-interactive world map with the marked places triggered a conversation. At least at this early stage in dementia it was easy for her to recognize the places on the map as places that were important in her life and she immediately started telling stories about them. The interactive map added the time dimension to this. When the time slider was set to a certain time period, Mrs Smith saw the places light up and referred to the time in the narratives. Given our experiences from the first two interviews with Mrs Smith, in which it was sometimes hard to match the stories to the correct timespans, the map supports remembering places and time. Similarly, Kalnikaite and colleagues [7] emphasized the value of locational information for aiding memories, and, in particular, for supporting inferences being made about past experiences.

6.2   Communication Points for Others

Equally important to the memory support for the person with dementia, we experienced ourselves the benefit of the interactive map in conversations with someone we know little about. One of the researchers who had not met Mrs Smith beforehand, could easily see on the map where Mrs Smith was born and which places she had visited at which times in her life. Especially in the case of places that the researcher had also lived in, it was easy to begin a conversation with Mrs Smith. It was also confirmed in the focus group that caregivers would use, for instance, recent holiday trips to start a conversation with residents, e.g., asking if they had been there. In this focus group, however, a wish for more advanced functionality was expressed as well. The idea of technology helping to find and visualize overlaps in several people's life stories was discussed and illustrated later on in the digital prototype.

6.3   Integration of Multimedia and Physical Artifacts

Existing multimedia systems already facilitate the sharing of stories and life events. They are, among others, available as online platforms, apps or other software. However, these are often not accessible to seniors, who are less technology savvy. Especially people with dementia have limited capacity to learn new interactions with digital user interfaces. Physical objects, however, provide at least three advantages: (1) interactions are based on familiar and basic actions (such as grabbing, moving or lifting objects), (2) they provide haptic stimulation, and (3) they often allow for shared interaction in a social setting. In our prototype we used the strength of both tangible interaction and multimedia content to provide a rich interface to cue reminiscence and allow for active use by people with dementia. In the user session with Mrs Smith, we could not observe any hesitation to use the interface. Instead Mrs Smith was curios about the map. We also did not have to provide lengthy explanations of how to operate the map.

In addition, the caregivers highlighted in the discussion about the digital extension of the system, that the tangible aspect of the prototype is important for the people with dementia. They suggested that the map could even have a more antique look and feel to it to trigger memories about maps used by the people in the past. For themselves, however, they preferred to have a system that offers more functional support for moderating a group session, e.g. by finding overlap of life events of several group members. Tangible interfaces, however, often work best if they have few functions, which are closely tight to the properties of the object. Therefore, to implement higher level functionality such as adding narrators and life events and comparing several narrators events, a digital interface was deemed more suited.

6.4 Equal Level Communication

Places provide a good means to trigger conversations with people with dementia, not simply because many people have visited the same places in their lives, but also because places are deeply intertwined with one's life story, which (1) allows residents to share their knowledge and (2) supports their life review. Keeping in mind that "[d]espite experiencing degeneration of short-term memory function, people with dementia (including individuals who are severely impaired) can very often retain a facility for long term memory that will function strongly given appropriate stimulation" [5], communication about their past should be possible for people with dementia until the later dementia stage.

As the care manager said in the focus group, an interactive map showing several people's places and stories, allows for a communication on an equal level between residents and caregivers. While people with dementia may have difficulties in taking part in conversations about everyday happenings or recent events, talking about important stories in their lives and discussing how places changed over time allows them to feel empowered. It puts emphasis on the vast experiences and knowledge that people of high age have. The interactive artefact would support the identification of interesting conversation topics between people, who, e.g., visited the same city or country at the same time or different times.

6.5 Leaving a Legacy

Closely linked to sharing one's life story with others is the aspect of leaving a legacy. For us, as designers of technology to support everyday life for people with dementia, Mrs Smith's reaction in the try-out session was rather surprising. While we expected the Reminiscence Map to be a tool for reminiscence for Mrs Smith herself, it became clear in the conversation that Mrs Smith was more concerned with preserving her life story for others after she cannot tell it herself anymore. Several times in the conversation she talked about placing the map in an exhibition for others to see or bequeathing it to someone she knows. She explicitly pointed out that it would be interesting for others to hear the stories, because she had travelled the world so much. While it remains unclear to us whether traveling the world was her own choice or simply a result of her life circumstances, her reflections on her life seemed to make her content and leaving her stories as a legacy beyond her own life span seemed important to her. Maybe it is especially important because she has few people left and no family of her own to continue telling her stories.

Important for the design of interactive artefacts, is to revise our assumptions of what is important for our target group and seeing the possibilities interactive technology can play in addressing their needs. While we assumed that communication in everyday life is an important need that technology should support, in this case, providing a means for casting one's experiences into an artefact that can be made accessible to others beyond one's life, surfaced as an important need, not in the first interviews, but in the session with the interactive prototype. Thus, the technology becomes a tool for a very different type of communication.

7 Limitations and Future Directions

Our work presents a single case study of how a need of a person with dementia was addressed in an interactive tangible artefact. This design case alone does not yet allow us to draw general conclusions about the role of advanced multimedia in supporting reminiscence in the large and diverse population of people with dementia. The themes, e.g. leaving a legacy, above are partially derived from data provided by a single person with dementia and it is, therefore, unclear if the same desire is present in other people. Yet, we believe this aspect is especially interesting to pursue in further research as it made us question our own design assumptions.

Arriving at a general theory on the design elements of interactive technologies for reminiscence and communication support is a longer term goal we pursue. As mentioned earlier other interactive artifacts have been developed and are being evaluated and discussed with similar sets of people in different care settings (for first results on that, see [6]). We see these artifacts more as boundary objects used to engage with stakeholders to understand their needs and discuss future possibilities. In this case, by making the idea of linking memories about life events to a time and place tangible in the two prototypes, they allowed us to explore the needs of the person deeper and discuss possibilities of advanced multimedia technologies with other stakeholders. As such the prototypes are vehicles to do research-through-design. Whether these or other designs truly have an effect on the level of reminiscence and foster communication of people with dementia needs to be studied in long-term field studies.

8   Conclusions

The work presented provides part of our larger research endeavour to design interactive multimedia artefacts for people with dementia to support their reminiscence and communication with others. In this paper we put the focus on one of the designed artefacts to show how this prototype could give us insights into the experiential world of a person with dementia and at the same time could be used in workshops and focus groups with experts as a probe triggering new ideas for designs in the care context. Especially the development of the second, digital prototype shows how the idea of linking memories to time and place was transformed and adapted to suit different stakeholders and use contexts. This way we could elicit views from different perspectives giving a more holistic picture of how the technology can support reminiscence and communication of people with dementia.

Besides this specific design case we are also field-testing several other designs (e.g. an interactive book, a virtual window to familiar places and a TV program for reminiscence). Based on the results of all evaluations, we intend to provide general guidelines for the design of interactive multimedia artefacts that support people with dementia in reminiscence and communication in different care settings. We should take into account that communication is manifold, and can also refer to communication beyond ones own life. In any case, the current case taught us to look carefully into the communication needs of people with dementia to check our own design assumptions.

Acknowledgements. We thank the students that have put their energy into doing field research in this sensitive area and developing the multimedia artifacts. Special thanks also go to all partners of the project from dementia care, technology development and related fields, who provided opportunities for field research and took part in workshops and focus groups providing helpful insights and feedback on our designs. Last, we thank all people with dementia and their caregivers for taking part in this research and opening up to us to share their life stories, concerns and wishes.

References

1. Alm, N., Astell, A., Gowans, G., Dye, R., Ellis, M., Vaughan, P., Riley, P.: Engaging multimedia leisure for people with dementia. Gerontechnology **8**(4), 236–246 (2009)
2. Astell, A., Alm, N., Gowans, G., Ellis, M., Dye, R., Vaughan, P.: Involving older people with dementia and their carers in designing computer based support systems: some methodological considerations. Univ. Access Inf. Soc. **8**(1), 49–58 (2009)
3. Ferri, C.P., Ames, D.: Behavioral and psychological symptoms of dementia in developing countries. Int. Psychogeriatr. **16**(04), 441–459 (2004)
4. Gallagher-Thompson, D., Tzuang, Y.M., Au, A., Brodaty, H., Charlesworth, G., Gupta, R., Lee, S.E., Losada, A., Shyu, Y.-I.: International perspectives on non-pharmacological best practices for dementia family caregivers: a review. Clin. Gerontologist **35**(4), 316–355 (2012)

5. Gowans, G., Campbell, J., Alm, N., Dye, R., Astell, A., Ellis, M.: Designing a multimedia conversation aid for reminiscence therapy in dementia care environments. In: CHI 2004 Extended Abstracts on Human Factors in Computing Systems, pp. 825–836. ACM (2004)
6. Huldtgren, A., Mertl, F., Vormann, A., Geiger, C.: Probing the potential of multimedia artefacts to support communication of people with dementia. In: Interact – The 15th IFIP TC 13 International Conference on Human-Computer Interaction, Bamberg, IFIP. ACM, September 2015
7. Kalnikaite, V., Sellen, A., Whittaker, S., Kirk, D.: Now let me see where i was: understanding how lifelogs mediate memory. In: Proceedings of the SIGCHI Conference on Human Factors in Computing Systems, pp. 2045–2054. ACM (2010)
8. Kasl-Godley, J., Gatz, M.: Psychosocial interventions for individuals with dementia: an integration of theory, therapy, and a clinical understanding of dementia. Clin. Psychol. Rev. **20**(6), 755–782 (2000)
9. Kitwood, T., Bredin, K.: Towards a theory of dementia care: personhood and wellbeing. Ageing Soc. **12**(03), 269–287 (1992)
10. Lazar, A., Thompson, H., Demiris, G.: A systematic review of the use of technology for reminiscence therapy. Health Educ. Behav. **41**(1 suppl), 51S–61S (2014)
11. Lindsay, S., Brittain, K., Jackson, D., Ladha, C., Ladha, K., Olivier, P.: Empathy, participatory design and people with dementia. In: Proceedings of the SIGCHI Conference on Human Factors in Computing Systems, pp. 521–530. ACM (2012)
12. Miskelly, F.: Electronic tracking of patients with dementia and wandering using mobile phone technology. Age Ageing **34**(5), 497–498 (2005)
13. Nilsson, M., Johansson, S., Håkansson, M.: Nostalgia: an evocative tangible interface for elderly users. In: CHI 2003 Extended Abstracts on Human Factors in Computing Systems, pp. 964–965. ACM (2003)
14. Orpwood, R., Bjørneby, S., Hagen, I., Mäki, O., Faulkner, R., Topo, P.: User involvement in dementia product development. Dementia **3**(3), 263–279 (2004)
15. Siriaraya, P., Ang, C.S.: Recreating living experiences from past memories through virtual worlds for people with dementia. In: Proceedings of the SIGCHI Conference on Human Factors in Computing Systems, pp. 3977–3986. ACM (2014)
16. Topo, P.: Technology studies to meet the needs of people with dementia and their caregivers a literature review. J. Appl. Gerontol. **28**(1), 5–37 (2009)
17. Wallace, J., Thieme, A., Wood, G., Schofield, G., Olivier, P.: Enabling self, intimacy and a sense of home in dementia: an enquiry into design in a hospital setting. In Proceedings of the SIGCHI Conference on Human Factors in Computing Systems, pp. 2629–2638. ACM (2012)
18. Wallace, J., Wright, P.C., McCarthy, J., Green, D.P., Thomas, J., Olivier, P.: A design-led inquiry into personhood in dementia. In: Proceedings of the SIGCHI Conference on Human Factors in Computing Systems, pp. 2617–2626. ACM (2013)
19. Waller, P.A., Östlund, B., Jönsson, B.: The extended television: using tangible computing to meet the needs of older persons at a nursing home. Gerontechnology **7**(1), 36–47 (2008)
20. Wood, W., Womack, J., Hooper, B.: Dying of boredom: an exploratory case study of time use, apparent affect, and routine activity situations on two alzheimer's special care units. Am. J. Occup. Ther. **63**(3), 337–350 (2009)
21. Woods, B., Portnoy, S., Head, D., Jones, G.: Reminiscence and life review with persons with dementia: which way forward. Care giving in dementia, pp. 137–161 (1992)

Interaction Model-Based User Interfaces: Two Approaches, One Goal - Comparison of Two User Interface Generation Approaches Applying Interaction Models

Miroslav Sili[✉], Matthias Gira, Markus Müllner-Rieder,
and Christopher Mayer

Health and Environment Department, Biomedical Systems,
AIT Austrian Institute of Technology GmbH, Vienna, Austria
{miroslav.sili,matthias.gira,markus.muellner-rieder,
christopher.mayer}@ait.ac.at

Abstract. Nowadays, we use a variety of devices to interact with local and cloud-based systems and services. We are accustomed to utilize an esthetic, functional and well-structured user interfaces. Most of these user interfaces are designed for the broad mass following the "one fits all" strategy. Undoubtedly, such a universal design approach has some benefits, but it has also some essential limitations. Inflexibility and the lack of possibilities for personalization are just two examples for these limitations. General designed user interfaces are not able to take specific user needs and requirements into account. Model-based user interface design tackles this challenge by creating abstract models which are used as starting point for the generation of tailored user interfaces. This work targets the comparison of two different interaction modeling techniques (CTT vs. SCXML) used for the design of multimodal user interfaces. Next to the general concepts, the corresponding execution frameworks and the practical exploration results are presented. The summary of elaborated advantages and disadvantages of each approach clarifies that the CTT approach is more applicable for large and complex user interaction scenarios, whereas the SCXML approach is more suitable for lightweight and structurally simpler user interaction scenarios.

Keywords: Interaction modeling · User interaction · Concurtasktrees · CTT · Statecharts · SCXML · Multimodality · Avatar based systems · Adaptivity

1 Introduction

Human Computer Interaction (HCI) and especially graphic based HCI is a widely discussed and still ongoing research area having its roots in the early 1970s. The desktop metaphor [1] presented by Xerox PARC on their very first computer with a Graphical User Interface (GUI) revolutionized the way how we interact with computers [2].

Compared to the previously widely used command based HCI methods, GUIs became more popular, because they are in general more intuitive, easier to understand

© Springer International Publishing Switzerland 2015
M. Helfert et al. (Eds.): ICT4AgeingWell 2015, CCIS 578, pp. 185–197, 2015.
DOI: 10.1007/978-3-319-27695-3_11

and simpler to use. However, these advantages came along with one significant disadvantage. GUI based applications require additional efforts in terms of time and costs for the design process. Therefore, researchers started to investigate new approaches to structure and to automate the design process. Work in this area ranged from design patterns like the Model Viewer Controller (MVC) [3], over different GUI builders and interface toolkits, to methods for an automatic generation of user interfaces based on an underlying data model [4–6].

Unfortunately, most of these user interface generation approaches were just applicable for a narrowly focused interface design. This early research became the foundation for model-based systems [7, 8]. Model-based systems exploit the idea of using a declarative model consisting of components such as user-task model, user model, dialog model, presentation model and domain model, in order to provide a formal representation of the user interface design [9].

This work compares two different user interaction modeling techniques used for the design of multimodal user interfaces. Interpretation engines for both techniques have been implemented in separate execution frameworks and both techniques have been evaluated in different Active Assisted Living (AAL) projects. User involvement results accomplished during the project trial phases are not in the scope of this paper and are separately published in [10].

In the beginning, we will provide a general overview about the two selected interaction modeling techniques (Sect. 2). The first is based on ConcurTaskTrees (CTT) [11] and the second is based on State Chart XML (SCXML) [12]. To be able to evaluate these interaction modeling techniques, we have developed two execution frameworks (Sect. 3). The first one reflects the prototype built within the project AALuis[1] and the second one reflects the prototype built within the project ibi[2]. By using these two prototypes, we are able to evaluate and to identify necessary tasks that user interaction developers need to fulfil in order to generate interaction models, to embed and connect these interaction models into the specific framework and finally to interpret them by using the runtime execution process. In Sect. 4, we provide a detailed comparison of advantages and disadvantages of the presented approaches based on eight evaluation categories. The comparison provides a clear identification of concrete use cases where each approach is superior to the other (Sect. 5).

2   Background

2.1   The CTT Interaction Model

CTT is an XML-based formal notation to represent task models. It is of hierarchical structure, with graphical syntax [13]. CTT focuses on activities to be executed by users or systems to reach a certain goal. CTT distinguishes between system, user, interaction, and abstract tasks. System tasks are executed by the (software) system alone (e.g., data processing). User tasks represent internal cognitive or physical activities performed by

---

[1] http://www.aaluis.eu.

[2] http://www.ibi.or.at.

the user of the system (e.g., selecting a problem solving strategy). Interaction tasks are user performed interactions with the system. Abstract tasks are used for composition of task groups in the hierarchical structure of the CTT. The notation provides an exhaustive set of temporal operators, which express the logical temporal relationships between the tasks.

Figure 1 illustrates a simple CTT model for the hotel room reservation scenario as published by the W3C Model-Based UI Working Group [14]. In the first step, the user is asked to select either a single room or a double room (represented by the two interaction tasks *SelectSingleRoom* and *SelectDoubleRoom*). In the second step, the system will provide a list of available rooms for the previously selected room type (represented by the *ShowAvailability* system task). In the third and last step, the user is asked to finally select one available room (represented by the *SelectRoom* interaction task). This example uses two types of temporal operators. First, the *choice* temporal operator to model a single selection between the two interaction tasks *SelectSingleRoom* and *SelectDoubleRoom*. And second, the *enabling with information passing* temporal operator to model a sequence, e.g., between the room selection and the reservation process.

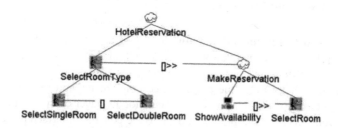

Fig. 1. Simple interaction model for the hotel room reservation scenario using the CTT

2.2   The Statechart Interaction Model

SCXML is an event-based state machine language [12]. It combines concepts from Harel State Tables [15] and Call Control eXtensible Markup Language (CCXML) [16, 17]. SCXML is widely used for user interfaces and dialog management in many different fields such as AAL, cloud based services or video games [18, 19]. It inherits semantics and special features like compound states and parallel states from Harel State Tables and combines it with event handling and the XML representation of CCXML. SCXML is used to describe Finite State Machines (FSM). A FSM is a mathematical model with a finite number of states where only one state can be active at any given time, called current state.

Figure 2 illustrates the interaction model of the hotel room reservation scenario using the SCXML notation. The initial state *SelectRoomType* has two transitions, namely *SelectSingleRoomType* and *SelectDoubleRoomType*. Depending on this first user choice the system will list either available single rooms or available double rooms. From the corresponding state the user has just one possibility to reach the final state *MakeReservation* by selecting one of the available rooms. This simplified example

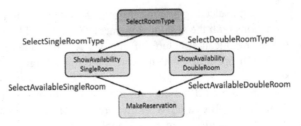

Fig. 2. Simple interaction model for the hotel room reservation scenario using the SCXML notation.

covers just a few tasks of a real hotel room reservation service, but it illustrates the main differences in interaction modelling using the CTT notation and the SCXML notation.

3   Execution Frameworks for Interaction Models

3.1   AAluis Execution Framework

Architecture and Communication Flow. The AALuis execution framework is an OSGi-based [20], flexible middleware layer. The framework dynamically generates user interfaces for connected services that provide CTT-modelled interaction descriptions [21]. Figure 3 illustrates the plugin-based components and the communication flow in the AALuis execution framework. The dialog manager component orchestrates the process from service description and data, to the concrete interface presented for a context specific interaction step. Service managers mediate between service endpoints and the dialog manager. Similarly, device managers act as brokers between the devices and the dialog manager.

The task description in CTT is the central document that services have to provide to the AALuis execution framework. It describes the interaction between the service and the user. For each interaction session, this component repeatedly evaluates the interaction

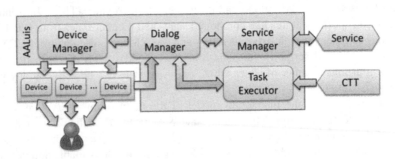

Fig. 3. Modules and communication flow in the AALuis execution framework.

status, generates and presents a user interface, applies user input, and re-evaluates the interaction status. The dialog manager is able to store interaction statuses of multiple service CTTs per session, but only one interaction can be in the foreground. Not only the dialog manager, but also the service itself can initiate an interaction. Through signaling of tasks of a certain type, the interaction flow is interrupted in a first-come-last-served manner.

The task execution component handles the run-time interpretation of the CTT by applying following execution steps. It (a) processes the current execution state of the CTT tree, (b) updates the state of one particular task, and (c) evaluates the CTT temporal operators to reach the new execution state. Based on these execution steps, the currently actable interaction tasks are used by the UI transformation component to generate a user interface.

Adoption of the standard rendering, and addition of new kinds of interaction, can be achieved in two ways: Either a completely new task-type is introduced into the CTT, or the interpretation of an existing type is redefined in the XSL files used for the transformation. Similarly, formerly unknown output modalities can be added to the execution framework. This entails using the new modality in the XSLT files. Output modalities and device types that are already registered can be included and excluded on-the-fly. The framework also provides the possibility for developers to create media conversion plug-in components that enable automatic conversion of one output modality to a new one.

Integration of CTT Interaction Models into the AALuis Execution Framework.
Next to the task description in CTT, services have to provide additionally a binding definition, associating the services' business methods to the tasks in the task description. These documents can be provided in two ways, depending on the residence of the service (external or internal).

External services are based on Web Service technology. They are not located in the AALuis framework itself nor deployed in the AAL middleware AALuis is deployed in. They are dynamically transformed and bound to an internal OSGi service representation, making them accessible by the framework. The CTT is provided by an URI that either points to a web resource or a local file. Internal services are based on OSGi technology. They have to be embedded into the same AAL middleware, and follow certain conventions. The OSGi bundle has to declare the bundle as AALuis service in the manifest and has to contain at least the above mentioned documents. Similar to external services a representation is created and used by the dialog manager. With these choices the service designer can concentrate efforts on the service and the planned interaction patterns alone. Encouraged by a very clear separation of concerns, the service designer does not need to think about the design of the elements that are forming the interaction, which is done independently by a UI designer.

New services can be integrated on-the-fly. Either by making the framework aware of a new external service endpoint or deployment of an internal OSGi bundle - also during runtime.

3.2   ibi Execution Framework

Architecture and Communication Flow. The ibi execution framework is a middleware, which connects different services with different in- and output modalities on various devices. These services and modalities can be exchanged and extended to create a tailored solution for a specific user and his/her set of services.

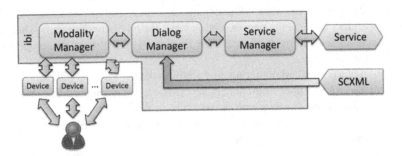

Fig. 4. Modules and communication flow in the ibi execution framework.

As depicted in Fig. 4, the system consists of the following main modules: the modality manager, the dialog manager and the service manager. The dialog manager is the central part of the ibi execution framework. It reads the SCXML definitions and parses them into internal SCXML dialog objects. Each dialog object represents a single statechart machine. The system supports multiple statechart machines which can be used concurrently. The dialog manager distributes all events received from the service manager or from the modality manager to all registered statechart machines. The service manager contains a list of registered services and sends requests from the dialog manager to the respective services. The modality manager has three main functionalities. First, it keeps track of all available devices and their modalities. Second, it is able to select either one specific or if needed multiple devices to deliver the required user interfaces. Third, it receives user inputs from the presented user interface and distributes them towards the dialog manager.

One of the main features of the ibi system is the possibility to address each single modality separately on each registered and available device, respectively. Thus, the system requires one device connector implementation for each new device type, e.g., one for Smartphones, one for TVs and one for PCs. Devices use these connectors to describe their available modalities to the system during the automatic device registration process, e.g., after a power up event. Analogous to this, each device requires also a concrete connector implementation on the device itself to be able to communicate with the ibi system. These implementations are already realized within the developed ibi client Apps for the smartphone, TV and PC device.

Each dialog object, respectively statechart, is connected to exactly one service. This one to one connection is used for the communication between the ibi system and the service. Transition triggers or state changes within the dialog object in the ibi system may cause an action on the service side and vice versa. Initially loaded dialog objects remain in their initial state until the first trigger event occurs. This event can be timer triggered, user input triggered or externally triggered (e.g., incoming event via HTTP). Moreover, dialog objects have a priority value. Dialogs with higher priority are able to interrupt lower priority dialogs, which are resumed when the high priority dialog finishes.

Integration of SCXMLs into the ibi Execution Framework. The service and an accompanying SCXML file have to be developed to integrate a new service into the ibi execution framework. The SCXML definitions are able to carry additional data within every state. In the ibi approach, this additional data fields are used to define special template-based treatments in the UI generation process. Templates may be defined, e.g., using XHTML [22] including XForms [23]. This allows customizing the generated user interfaces if needed. Unfortunately this practical feature has also one disadvantage. In the current implementation new template types require also new interpreters in form of source code implementations within the execution framework. This blurs the responsibilities between two parties because neither the service designers (who generate SCXMLs), nor the UI designers (who generate templates and their implementations) should be forced to modify and extend the framework. As a future improvement the ibi approach requires a new strategy to support new templates without the need to extend the framework by additional implementations.

In the ibi approach a service can be created either as internal or external service. Internal services are integrated into the ibi execution framework, while external services interact via Representational State Transfer (REST) calls [24]. To accomplish this, an external service manager is implemented as an abstraction layer between the external service and the service manager. This abstraction allows external services to register themselves as internal services, which facilitates a consistent access.

3.3   Examples of Generated Uis

Figures 5 and 6 illustrate examples of generated User Interfaces for the TV device. Figure 5 illustrates a reminder service where current user's appointments are visualized. Figure 6 illustrates a simple messaging service where the user is asked to choose one out of three possible messages to be sent to his or her relatives. Both approaches use avatars as additional modality to support the user. The TV device implementations in both approaches support a remote control based navigation. While the AALuis approach is limited to an arrow based navigation (up, down, left, right), the ibi approach supports additionally the number based navigation.

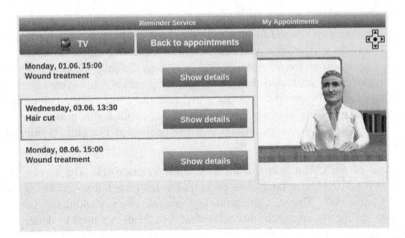

Fig. 5. Sample TV user interface generated by the AALuis approach visualizing a reminder service.

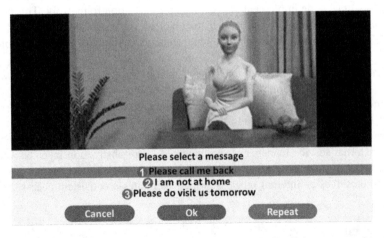

Fig. 6. Sample TV user interface generated by the ibi approach visualizing a messaging service.

4   Results

This chapter provides a comparison of advantages and disadvantages of the presented approaches based on the following eight evaluation categories: (a) generation of the interaction model, (b) UI customization and UI extensibility, (c) concurrency, (d) separation of concerns, (e) modality and device extensibility, (f) integration of new services, (g) tool for the interaction design, and finally (h) modality conversion and alternative modalities. The comparison focuses on applicability aspects from the technical point of view.

4.1 Detailed Comparison

Generation of the Interaction Model. The interaction model in the AALuis approach is able to generate complex interaction scenarios. The CTT notation provides a high degree of flexibility using temporal operators allowing task processing in different orders, e.g., sequential, concurrent or interrupting. Unfortunately, this flexibility requires additional efforts when learning the CTT notation.

In contrast, the SCXML interaction model in the ibi approach is easier to learn. It is composed by just two elements, namely states and transitions. The disadvantage of this simplicity is the limitation when modelling complex interactions. Developers need to define numerous transitions between single states to compensate missing constructs for concurrency and interruption. This makes the system impracticable for rich interaction scenarios.

UI Customization and UI Extensibility. In the AALuis approach, a new UI element (e.g., a calendar widget or captions) is created by defining a new task type in the interaction model. The framework transforms this new task type into an abstract XML element which is finally rendered using XSL rules. Both extensions, the definition of the new task type as well as the XSL rules, can be defined independently and outside of the AALuis framework. This allows extensibility which does not require to rebuild or to recompile the AALuis framework.

In the ibi prototype, UI customization is achieved by defining new templates within the interaction model. These templates are filled with concrete data during the final rendering process. The framework supports the interpretation of different templates but it is limited in the generation of new UI elements. Interpretations of new template types require new implementations, which also imply the rebuilding of the ibi framework.

Concurrency. The AALuis framework supports concurrent interaction models, which allow multiple user-system interaction dialogs. The current implementation is limited in prioritization of these concurrent interaction models. Because each dialog owns the same priority level, the framework is not able to distinguish between more important dialogs (e.g., security warnings) and less important dialogs (e.g., incoming social network messages). To overcome this ambiguity, the priority responsibility in the AALuis approach is shifted to the service side. The service has to decide which dialog is prioritized higher and which dialog has to be postponed due its low level priority.

The ibi approach supports concurrent interaction models and different priority levels. Each interaction model is clearly assigned to a priority level. High priority dialogs are able to interrupt low priority dialogs. These are resumed once the higher priority level dialogs are finished. Dialogs with the same priority level are served in the First In First Out (FIFO) order.

Separation of Concerns. The separation of concerns is clearly achieved in the AALuis approach. UI designers, on the one hand, are responsible for extending and maintaining XSL rules for new UI elements, new branding styles and new device types. Service designers, on the other hand, are responsible for defining, maintaining and connecting their services. Therefore, UI designers do not need to be involved during the service integration and oppositely service designers do not need to take care about UI related topics.

The ibi approach has blurred responsibilities between service and UI designers. Extensions on both sides require to rebuild and to recompile the ibi framework, respectively. Therefore, the UI designer is not able to extend the framework without the explicit involvement of the service designer and vice versa.

Modality and Device Extensibility. Both systems are able to keep track of available and connected devices and modalities, but the extensibility is handled in a different manner. In the AALuis prototype, new modalities are included by applying new XSL transformations. In some cases, these new modalities require also new devices (e.g., modality for Braille lettering). These devices can be included and/or excluded on the fly, because AALuis-enabled devices are able to automatically describe their capabilities towards the AALuis framework. Furthermore, the framework has a complete overview about available and connected devices. A concrete device can be addressed, depending on the required modality.

In the ibi approach, new device types are not able to describe themselves automatically. Each new device type requires a connection in form of a concrete source code implementation on the framework side. Once this work is done, the framework will be able to address the specific connected device type depending on the required modality.

Integration of New Services. The AALuis prototype is able to dynamically connect SOAP-based external and OSGi-based internal services. Therefore, service designers do not need to extend the framework in form of new source code implementations.

New services in the ibi approach require a concrete source code implementation. As a result of this new implementation, the whole framework has to be rebuilt. New implementations are not restricted to a specific communication method. A lightweight and easy to deploy REST-based communication method can be used in the ibi approach.

Tool for the Interaction Design. For both prototypes external graphical tools can be used to design the interaction model. The CTTE-tool [25] used in the AALuis approach has a built-in simulator, which allows an early pretesting of the interaction model.

The graphical tool scxmlgui [26] used in the ibi prototype does not provide a simulator. Considering the lightweight complexity of SCXML elements (states and transitions) a simulator would not be able to provide more information than the design tool.

Modality Conversion and Alternative Modalities. An avatar-based user-system interaction was one of the main requirements in both projects. Therefore, both approaches have a built-in text to avatar modality conversion. Besides, both systems do not support an additional automatic modality conversion currently. The AALuis prototype supports alternative modalities (e.g., a textual representation of an image) but these alternative elements need to be provided by the service.

4.2   Summary of Evaluation Results

Table 1 summarizes the evaluated advantages and disadvantages of the presented techniques and provides a comparison between them. Positive aspects are marked with a '+' sign, neutral aspects are marked with a 'o' sign and negative aspects are marked with a '−' sign.

Table 1. Comparison between the current status of the AALuis and the ibi approach (legend: +..positive aspect, o..neutral aspect, −..negative aspect).

	AALuis/CTT	ibi/SCXML
Generation of the interaction model	+ Supports the generation of complex interaction scenarios − Efforts needed to learn the CTT notation	− Limitations in the complexity + Easy to understand and easy to learn
UI customization and UI extensibility	+ Supports the definition of new task types and therefore new UI elements + Supports new task type interpretations by external XSL rules	+ Supports template definitions within every state − Interpretations of new templates require new implementations
Concurrency	o Framework supports concurrency of multiple CTTs but without a prioritization of interactions	+ Framework supports concurrency of multiple SCXMLs and priority definitions
Separation of concerns	+ Clear separation between service designers and UI designers	− Blurred responsibilities between service designers and UI designers
Modality and device extensibility	o New modalities require new XSL transformation rules + Devices and modalities may be included and/or excluded on the fly	− New modalities require new implementations − New devices require new implementations
New service integration	+ New services can be integrated on-the-fly + Support of internal or external SOAP based web service	− New services require new implementations + Support of internal or external REST based web service
Tool for the interaction design	+ GUI for the design of CTTs + Simulator allows an early pretesting	+ GUI for the design of SCXMLs o Simulation and pre-testings are not possible
Multimodality conversion and alternative modalities	+ Built-in text to avatar modality conversion + Support for alternative modalities	+ Built-in text to avatar modality conversion − New modality conversions require new implementations

5 Conclusions

In this work, two different interaction modeling techniques, the corresponding execution frameworks and the practical exploration results from the technical point of view have been presented. The comparison of the exploration results clarifies that the CTT approach applied in AALuis is more applicable for large and complex user interaction scenarios. The SCXML approach applied in the ibi project is more suitable for lightweight and structurally simpler user interaction scenarios.

Although the proposed techniques and execution frameworks already provide beneficial and useable results, we expect to improve both systems. In the AALuis approach, we intend to focus on a semi-automatic generation of CTT models. Introducing some kind of prioritization on service or task-group level would conceivably mitigate the shortcomings of the concurrent execution of the interactions. In the ibi approach, we intend to focus on a semi-automatic binding between the SCXML states and external services. Another improvement for ibi would be the automatic generation of modality specific output without the need of a concrete implementation for the template interpretation.

Acknowledgements. The project AALuis was co-funded by the AAL Joint Programme (REF. AAL-2010-3-070) and the following National Authorities and R&D programs in Austria, Germany and The Netherlands: BMVIT, program benefit, FFG (AT), BMBF (DE) and ZonMw (NL).

The ibi project was co-funded by the benefit programme of the Federal Ministry for Transport, Innovation and Technology (BMVIT) of Austria.

References

1. Smith, D.C., et al.: The desktop metaphor as an approach to user interface design (panel discussion). In: Proceedings of the 1985 ACM Annual Conference on the Range of Computing: mid-80's Perspective: mid-80's Perspective, pp. 548–549 (1985)
2. Thacker, C.P., et al.: Alto: A personal computer. Xerox Palo Alto Research Center, Report CSL-79-11, vol. 445 (1979)
3. Burbeck, S.: Applications programming in smalltalk-80 (tm): How to use model-view-controller (mvc)., Smalltalk-80 v2.5 (1992)
4. Krasner, G.E., et al.: A description of the model-view-controller user interface paradigm in the smalltalk-80 system. J. Object Oriented Program. 1(3), 26–49 (1988)
5. Janssen, C., et al.: Generating user interfaces from data models and dialogue net specifications. In: Proceedings of the INTERACT 1993 and CHI 1993 Conference on Human Factors in Computing Systems, pp. 418–423 (1993)
6. De Baar, D., et al.: Coupling application design and user interface design. In: Proceedings of the SIGCHI Conference on Human Factors in Computing Systems, pp. 259–266 (1992)
7. Puerta, A.R., et al.: Model-based automated generation of user interfaces. In: AAAI, pp. 471–477 (1994)
8. Puerta, A.R., et al.: Towards a general computational framework for model-based interface development systems. Knowl. Based Syst. 12(8), 433–442 (1999)

9. Puerta, A.R.: A model-based interface development environment. IEEE Softw. **14**(4), 40–47 (1997)
10. Sili, M., Bobeth, J., Sandner, E., Hanke, S., Schwarz, S., Mayer, C.: Talking faces in lab and field trials. In: Zhou, J., Salvendy, G. (eds.) ITAP 2015. LNCS, vol. 9193, pp. 134–144. Springer, Heidelberg (2015)
11. Paternò, F., et al.: ConcurTaskTrees: A diagrammatic notation for specifying task models. In: Human-Computer Interaction INTERACT 1997, pp. 362–369 (1997)
12. Barnett, J., et al.: State Chart XML (SCXML): State machine notation for control abstraction, W3C working draft (2007)
13. Paternò, F.: Concur task trees: an engineered notation for task models. In: The Handbook of Task Analysis for Human-Computer Interaction, pp. 483–503 (2003)
14. Paternò, F., et al.: W3C MBUI - Task Models. http://www.w3.org/TR/2012/WD-task-models-20120802/. Accessed 28 September 2015
15. Harel, D.: Statecharts: a visual formalism for complex systems. Sci. Comput. Program. **8**(3), 231–274 (1987)
16. Auburn, R.J., et al.: Voice browser call control: CCXML version 1.0, W3C Working Draft (2005)
17. Romellini, C., et al.: CCXML: The Power of Standardization. Loquendo, Turin (2005)
18. Dragert, C.: Model-Driven Development of AI for Digital Games, Diss. McGill University (2013)
19. Jeong, H., et al.: Multimodal Interface for Mobile Cloud Computing. Latest Advances in Information Science and Applications, pp. 270–274. WSEAS Press, Venice (2012)
20. Alliance, O.: OSGi service platform, release 3. IOS Press, Inc., Amsterdam (2003)
21. Mayer, C., et al.: A comparative study of systems for the design of flexible user interfaces. J. Ambient Intell. Smart Environ. (2015, in press/accepted)
22. Pemberton, S.: XHTML™ 1.0 the extensible hypertext markup language. W3C Recommendations, pp. 1–11 (2000)
23. Boyer, J.M., et al.: XForms 1.1, W3C Recommendation 20 (2009)
24. Richardson, L., et al.: RESTful web services. O'Reilly Media, Inc., Sebastopol (2008)
25. Mori, G., et al.: CTTE: support for developing and analyzing task models for interactive system design. IEEE Trans. Softw. Eng. **28**(8), 797–813 (2002)
26. Code.google.com, scxmlgui - A graphical editor for SCXML finite state machines.- Google Project Hosting. https://code.google.com/p/scxmlgui/. Accessed 28 September 2015

Older Adults Digital Gameplay: A Follow-up Study of Social Benefits

Simone Hausknecht[✉], Robyn Schell, Fan Zhang, and David Kaufman

Faculty of Education, Simon Fraser University, Burnaby, Canada
{shauskne,rmschell,fza26,dkaufman}@sfu.ca

Abstract. This study involved 20 Wii Bowling teams of 3–4 players each in an eight-week tournament across a large city in western Canada. This paper summarizes the initial results, in which an increase in social connectedness and decrease in loneliness were found, and reports on a follow-up study three months after the tournament that examined whether people still played together and maintained their social connections. The follow-up consisted of 14 focus groups, with 46 Wii Bowling players, with at least one representative from each team. Many participants seemed to maintain benefit from their new social contacts three months after the tournament. However, participants experienced some difficulties in recruiting new players and in maintaining momentum over time. In seniors' centres and facilities with scheduled activities, Wii Bowling remained a regular source of social interaction and fun. These findings are examined with a consideration of socio-emotional selectivity theory.

Keywords: Aging · Digital games · Loneliness · Motivation · Older adults · Social connectedness · Videogames

1 Introduction

1.1 Background

It is estimated that from 2010 to 2050, the older demographic (65+) will triple in population, creating a disproportionate number of people in this age group compared to other groups [1]. The growth of the older adult population has led to an increased focus on what this means for society and for this age group. Aging can involve changes such as declines in cognitive and physical abilities and altered relationships, social contacts, lifestyle, and living conditions [2]. Older adults face increased concerns about issues such as fractures, cognitive decline, and isolation that may affect day to day living [3]. The demographic change will have both positive and negative impacts on institutions, work places, culture, and society, as efforts increase to help older adults enjoy fulfilling and productive lives and to maintain their quality of life [3–5].

Quality of life has many components, often including some level of socio-emotional, physical, functional, and cognitive wellbeing [5, 6]. To further these ideas, the United Nations and the World Health Organization have helped to popularize discussions of 'active aging' as a goal [7]. Active aging can be defined as "the process of optimizing opportunities for health, participation and security in order to enhance quality of life as

© Springer International Publishing Switzerland 2015
M. Helfert et al. (Eds.): ICT4AgeingWell 2015, CCIS 578, pp. 198–216, 2015.
DOI: 10.1007/978-3-319-27695-3_12

people age" [3]. An international call for research on an aging society attempts to create an atmosphere in which people can age well [7].

Social relationships and contacts in a person's life are an important component of aging well and are influential in a variety of ways. Social interactions influence life trajectories and health outcomes spanning across physical [8], cognitive [9], and general wellbeing [10].

As people age, their relationships and social networks often change. Older adults tend to have smaller but more meaningful networks than younger adults [11]. However, they may lack social connectedness, or a sense of belonging, at various times. If their social connections are suddenly disrupted (e.g., by death, moving, or other events), individuals can find themselves becoming isolated. Leisure activities may be a way to increase social connections [12].

In recent years, interest has increased in using digital games for enhancing the lives of older adults, and researchers have explored their possible cognitive, emotional, physical, and social benefits [13, 14]. Games can help to motivate older adults and can contribute to specific improvements in their quality of life [15]. Digital games may provide a social context in which new relationships and connections can form. Designs of digital games for older adults have often considered this, and researchers have identified both socializing and interacting as important [16]. Although some studies have found that digital games provide an opportunity to increase social interactions and possibly decrease loneliness (e.g. [17–19]), further examination and in-depth study would be useful, in particular by examining whether the playful medium of a digital game can create a positive emotional experience that facilitates social connections. Determining the nature of these relationships and whether they have the potential for longevity is important.

It is also important to determine whether an intervention is sustained after the research has been conducted. Past research on sustainability of interventions suggests that results do not always continue when a study has finished [20]. Games within themselves can be motivational, but the ability to sustain activities afterwards might be difficult even though participants are engaged during a tournament. Furthermore, if social connections are made, do these continue afterwards and remain a part of the individual's social network?

This paper summarizes the initial socio-emotional results of a Wii Bowling tournament [21, 22] and expands on these by presenting the results of a follow-up study that examined further Wii Bowling use and experience three months after the intervention.

1.2 Purpose of the Study

The purpose of the earlier study was to determine whether a digital game was effective in enhancing various socio-emotional conditions including social connectedness and loneliness. The purpose of the current paper is to report on a follow-up study to determine (1) how participants perceived and experienced the social aspects of the game three months after the tournament ended, and (2) whether they continued to play. Thus, it studied whether the game itself created a sustainable, self-motivating environment, or whether further intervention would be required.

2   Literature Review

2.1   Social Connectedness, Loneliness, and Socioemotional Selectivity Theory

Interacting and feeling socially connected are essential parts of our experiences throughout the life span. These connections and the interactions we have with others can influence further life trajectories [23]. A person does not exist as an isolated member of society no matter how little contact they have with others. The need for social interactions is important at all age groups. Beaumeister and Leary [24] suggest that belonging is an essential human need; we form attachments easily and often don't let them go easily. They argue that the need for belonging is one of the main drives that makes us seek out relationships, particularly those that are positive and lasting. For the older adult, social connections and engagement can be a major contributor to their quality of life and sense of wellbeing [5, 10, 25].

Other authors have reported that social connections and engagement are important for wellbeing, and can contribute to improved health outcomes [8, 26, 27]. For example, one study showed that social activities were effective in maintaining wellbeing and a positive mental state and social contacts and relationships had positive outcomes for health [8]. Glei et al. [9] found that cognition was related to social engagement and network size; study participants who took part in more social activities performed better on cognitive tests than those that had had fewer or none. Furthermore, they suggested that social networks outside the family might increase cognitive abilities, compared to within the family. A survey in Europe of 26,788 adults over 50 years of age discovered that social participation increased self-reported health outcomes [27]. This may also form a protective mechanism for various disorders such as dementia [28].

The importance of social interactions can be examined in a variety of ways. It could be seen through the lens of value (social capital), aid (social support), structure, ties, diversity of contacts (social network), and perceptions of belonging (social connectedness). However, all of these influence each other. Social capital can be seen as the resources and benefits available to a person through their social connections [29]. This has been found to affect older adults in a variety of ways, including their sense of wellbeing [10]. However, social capital can depend on a person's social network and the types of connections that they have. At times, more diverse connections are more beneficial [30].

These connections may fulfil different needs, such as social support or a sense of social connectedness. Social connectedness can be defined as a person's feelings of belonging and being able to relate to others [31]. While social support is often seen as serving a helping role, social connectedness does not need to do so. Social support does not necessarily fulfil the role of belonging [26]. Social connectedness may simply come from casual leisure relationships and companionship; it allows for the enjoyment of another's company, thus fulfilling a social need [26]. Social connectedness, i.e., belonging, serves a valuable purpose in the life course of the individual and their wellbeing. Furthermore, a person's sense of belonging may be one of the main social factors that influence the extent to which a person finds life meaningful [32].

Lack of social connectedness can be intimately related to loneliness [33]. Without a feeling of belonging and being socially connected, a person may become isolated and feelings of loneliness may arise [34]. Loneliness can be described as a disturbing sensation that arises when a person perceives that their social needs are not being met by their social connections [35]. Hawksley and Cacioppo [35] suggest that because this is a perception, people can be alone but not feel lonely.

Research on whether older adults have an increased chance of loneliness has shown mixed results. Pinquart and Sorensen [36] conducted a meta-analysis in which they found that adults over the age of 80 were more likely to report increased loneliness. Dykstra, van Tilberg and de Jong Gierveld [37] conducted a longitudinal study in which they found that loneliness scores increased for older adults over time. Interestingly, they found that when older adults' social networks increased, their feelings of loneliness decreased, suggesting that simply increasing contacts may have an effect.

Social networks are the web of relationships and individual connections one has in their life [26]. They incorporate numerous groups from family, acquaintances, neighbours, friends, and community and are the contextual basis in which interactions and perceptions of connection occur [26]. In theory, forming networks may be a good place to begin to increase social connectedness [31]. Often the more social ties a person has, the more socially connected they feel [38]. However, it has been suggested that older adults often have smaller social networks and fewer connections by choice [11].

Motivation for social interactions and forming new social connections may change throughout the lifespan. In socio-emotional selectivity theory (SST), Carstensen [11] suggests that later in life we selectively limit our relationships. This is partly due to an increasing sense that time is limited, so that forming new relationships may not seem as worthwhile as maintaining established ones. Furthermore, a person who is young and exploring self-concept will have increased social networks and contacts that challenge identity, whereas a person who is older tends to prefer social relationships that will reaffirm who they are. Novel social partners may create a threat to this. Older adults are often motivated by emotional benefit, so that social contacts are based on affective qualities [11]. This is due to emotional regulation, an important competence in later life. However, older adults often find leisure activities to be more rewarding within a social context [39].

Because older adults are more likely to select social relationships that are familiar rather than novel [11, 40], leisure activity aiming to increase social connections may require a period of time to establish familiarity and build strong ties. Many older adults seek out leisure activities within a social context [39]. Although family and close friends may be seen as older adults' most important and worthwhile relationships, those that come about through enjoyable leisure activities and shared experience are also important, especially in retirement villages where there is regular contact with neighbours [12]. This may be related to ideas of the benefits of social connectedness and the immediate gratification of belonging to a group. Leisure activities are beneficial without taking too many extra resources if they are enjoyable and social to begin with.

Researchers have argued that efforts to increase social connectedness through leisure activity should incorporate emotional appeal. Technology may provide a medium for social connections and entertainment [41]. In particular, digital games can create fun, challenging environments where older adults can socialize and share positive emotional experiences.

2.2 Digital Games and Older Adults

Digital games are being increasingly examined as possible tools and platforms to enhance older adults' quality of life [15, 16]. Studies have found that digital games can provide physical, social, emotional, and cognitive benefits that may contribute to well-being.

Older adults are increasingly becoming gamers. In 2014, 27 % of older adult gamers were over age 50 [42]. Furthermore, the number of female gamers age 50 and older increased by 32 % from 2012 to 2013 [43]. Older adults are often consistent, regular users once they start playing [44, 45]. De Schutter [17] found that social interaction was one of the main predictors of older adults' consumption time within a game.

The use of digital games for entertainment, to pass the time, or for fun is not surprising [46]. Nimrod [47] found that older adults in an online forum were there mainly for fun, in what he described as a "fun culture." However, given the subjectiveness of the word, defining "fun" is difficult. When related to digital games, it is often mixed with challenge, engagement, and flow. Flow creates a sense of satisfaction from an immersive activity where a person is so absorbed that they lose track of time [48]. In a game environment, it is often created through challenge-based pleasure [49]. Challenge and enjoyment have often been seen as two of the main motivations for gameplay [17, 46]. A recent qualitative study of 15 participants suggested that exergames (in this study, the X-box 360 Kinect) satisfied the psychological needs of autonomy and competence that are required for self-regulation [50]. The importance of autonomy (the freedom to perform an activity), and competence (the actual ability to do so) may be particularly important for new players. However, it has been argued that social interaction is also a motivating force for gameplay [15]. Gamberini et al. [51] suggested that, in their Elder-games project, creating connections and facilitating social interactions were significant benefits.

Wii games have been used in a number of studies with older adults and have shown some benefits (e.g., see [18, 19, 52]). Using Wii games to improve balance and exercise has shown positive results [53]. Exergames have also shown promise for rehabilitation and prevention [54], for improving psychological health [19], and for increasing overall wellbeing [52]. Jung et al. [52] noted that senior centres play an important role in encouraging older adults to use new technologies.

Many digital games provide a medium for play with others, either competitively or collaboratively, that can increase social interactions. For example, a study involving 35 older adults who either watched TV or played Wii games, found that the Wii group had a more positive mood and lower levels of loneliness [18]. An intervention study found that after playing Wii games together in a community dwelling, older adults reported that gameplay had increased their bonding with other players [19]. Furthermore, game-play has been reported as helpful for reducing feelings of loneliness [17].

The potential of digital games for increasing social interaction is not limited to the actual gameplay. Discussing games within social networks has also been shown to provide opportunities to exchange information and have fun socializing [55, 56]. Nimrod [55] found that older adults used an online social website to satisfy their need for play while fostering communication and community.

As shown above, previous studies of older adults' digital gameplay have had successful outcomes. However, very few have examined whether motivation to play, social interactions, and gameplay benefits are sustained in the longer term.

3 Research Questions

This study was guided by the following questions:

1. When socio-emotional benefits are perceived by older adults after a digital game intervention, do these benefits continue afterwards?
2. What are the social experiences three months later of older adults who participated in an eight-week Wii Bowling tournament?
3. Is playing the Wii Bowling digital game sustainable after the intervention?

4 Research Method

This study investigated outcomes of a Wii Bowling tournament for older adults held over a two-month period. The Wii digital bowling game was chosen because it allows for multiple players and is reasonably accessible to older age groups. Furthermore, many older adults are familiar with bowling. The tournament utilized both collaboration (participants played in teams) and competition (teams competed for cash rewards). Data were collected with pre- and post-tournament questionnaires, post-tournament interviews, focus groups after three months, and a brief one-year follow-up telephone survey.

4.1 Recruitment

Initially, a number of seniors' centres in the Greater Vancouver, Canada area were approached to help recruit participants and to provide space for gameplay. In total, 14 centres participated. Posters and flyers were used to recruit participants, advertising dates for information sessions with a researcher to explain the study and tournament in detail. After these sessions, 20 teams were formed. Three months after the tournament, centres helped to contact and recruit 46 tournament participants for focus groups.

4.2 Participants

Participants consisted of 73 adults aged 65 and over from 14 different centres, including independent living centres, senior recreation centres, and assisted living complexes where participants either lived or frequently visited. Seventeen of the participants volunteered to take part in the in-depth post-tournament interview. Forty-six participants, including at least one representative from each team and from each centre, participated in the three-month follow-up focus groups. After one year, centre facilitators or social coordinators participated in brief phone follow-up interviews

4.3 Data Collection and Instruments

The study used a mixed methods approach with both questionnaires and semi-structured interviews to collect the data. This allowed for a triangulation of the results, helping to confirm the findings while also allowing us to dive deeper into the participants' experience.

First, pre- and post-tournament questionnaires were given to all participants. These included background/demographics such as age, sex, living arrangements; levels of loneliness and social isolation; and attitudes toward video games. The questionnaires were adapted from the UCLA Loneliness Scale [57] and the Overall Social Connectedness Dimensions [31]. The adaption included rewording to make all the statement forms and response scales consistent. A group of researchers then tested each sentence for understanding, and where there was confusion the phrasing was altered for clarity. The response scale options were "strongly disagree," "disagree," "unsure," "agree," and "strongly agree." Respondents required 15–20 min to complete the survey and received a $20 honorarium for completing each questionnaire.

Pre- and post- semi-structured interviews were conducted for 17 participants. The second interview was based on semi-structured questions that asked about participants' perceptions of their game experience during the tournament. This allowed the researchers to develop a more in-depth understanding of the participants' experience with the game and the connections they made during the tournament.

For the three-month follow-up study, focus groups were formed and semi-structured interviews (10 min) were conducted by a research assistant. Each participant from the focus group received a $5 gift card for their participation. After one year, a research assistant held final phone interviews with centre facilities co-ordinators or managers to determine if and to what extent the Wii was still being used.

4.4 Data Analysis

Quantitative data analysis was done using SPSS v. 21.0. Demographics were examined using frequencies and percentages, and paired sample t-tests were conducted comparing pre-test and post-test scores on social connectedness and loneliness.

The interviews were transcribed and then analyzed to find common codes. MaxQDA software was used to help with the coding. Codes were collected and major themes identified. Only those codes that were present in at least 50 % of the interviews were examined for overarching themes, one of which was social connectedness.

The follow-up interviews were also transcribed and then analyzed for common codes. Once again these were examined for overarching themes. Finally, all transcripts were searched for the word "fun" to identify additional themes related to enjoyment.

5 Findings

The quantitative and qualitative findings for the study are reported below.

5.1 Participants' Backgrounds

Frequencies and percentages for participants' background characteristics are summarized in Table 1. A higher proportion of participants (almost three quarters) were female, compared to males. Participants' ages were fairly evenly distributed, with over one third aged 85 or over. Approximately two thirds of participants lived alone versus only one third living with another person, and half were in assisted or independent living situations.

Table 1. Participant background characteristics.

Characteristics	Category	Frequency (N)	Percent (%)
Sex	Male	21	28.8
	Female	52	71.2
	Total	73	100
Age	65–74	21	28.8
	75–84	27	37
	85+	25	34.2
	Total	73	100
Living arrangement	Alone	51	69.9
	Other	22	30.1
	Total	73	100
Housing	House	7	9.6
	Condo	29	39.7
	Independent/Assisted living	37	50.7
	Total	73	100

5.2 Social Connectedness

A paired-samples t-test was conducted to compare social connectedness before and after the tournament (Table 2). There was a significant increase ($t(72) = 2.18$, $p = 0.033$) in social connectedness scores before ($M = 3.410$, $SD = 0.528$) and after gameplay ($M = 3.526$, $SD = 0.485$). This suggests that the two months of game playing increased participants' social connectedness.

Table 2. Paired samples t-test comparing pre-test and post-test scores on social connectedness.

Group	Pre-test mean (SD)	Post-test mean (SD)	Effect size	t	p
(N = 73)	3.41 (0.53)	3.53 (0.49)	0.42	2.18	.033

5.3   Loneliness

Table 3 shows the results of a paired samples t-test test comparing pre-test and post-test scores on loneliness. There was a significant difference (t (70) = 3.518, p = 0.001) in the scores before (M = 2.214, SD = 0.528) and after (M = 2.049, SD = 0.54) the two-month tournament.

Table 3. Paired samples t-tests comparing pre-test and post-test scores on loneliness.

Group	Pre-test mean (SD)	Post-test mean (SD)	Effect size	t	p
(N = 71)	2.21 (0.53)	2.05 (0.54)	0.42	3.52	.001

5.4   Social Connectedness as Reflected in Individual Interviews and Focus Groups

Qualitative data analysis of the 17 interview transcripts revealed an overarching theme of increased social connectedness from playing Wii Bowling [21, 22]. This was also found in the focus group interviews. Table 4 combines these results, since similar codes were found for both. However, only two were relevant (with over 50 % reporting the code) for both the initial interviews and focus groups and thus consistent over the three-month time frame. (For a more in-depth discussion on the interview results, see [22]. Although the focus group interviews were much shorter and focused on the three months after the tournament, the focus group participants still spoke about the tournament. Codes that were specifically talking about their social interactions since the tournament were separated, and a new code was defined for continued connections (see Table 4).

Table 4. Number of times and participants that a code was found.

| Code | Interviews | | Focus group | |
	No. of times applied	No. of participants	No. of times applied	No. of groups
Increased interactions	84	16	18	9
Stronger social connections	70	13	15	7
Continued connections	N/A	N/A	18	9

Social connectedness continued as a major theme three months after the tournament. The following sections describe comments from both the initial interviews and follow-up focus groups on increased social interactions and stronger social connections, providing some insights on the continuity of these benefits over time. Continued connections are discussed separately below.

Increased Social Interactions. During the interviews and focus groups, participants commented on how the intervention had increased their social interactions. The enjoyable environment had allowed for a relaxed way to interact with each other. As this focus group participant stated, "It was just fun, us together was fun. It makes you more comfortable – you know more people." An interview participant seemed to share this sentiment, reporting that:

> I would say my spirits have been uplifted a bit. Definitely, and it's because of this activity. Because up to that point in time, I just do my thing and go about my daily business, so to speak. But this, again, brought us together and [was] very beneficial.

Some interactions continued outside of the game. For example, as one participant, pointed out:

> Well, I got to know the lady next door. And because she was on my team, and we found out that we lived next door to each other. So we are going to share a garden spot together. Um, and now that I look at the size of the spot, we probably both needed one. But anyway, we will garden together. We're going to buy the plants together. So, yes, I met my neighbour. So that was—and I might not have spent the time with her otherwise.

For one participant, this opportunity to get to know people and get together with them on a regular basis was important to belonging. She stated that "you get to associate with people you probably wouldn't normally associate with all the time, and it gives you a sense of belonging, right."

These interactions were not limited to the tournament players. They also included others who came to watch the team play because, as one player noted, "we had people come to watch. Because they showed interest, they thought 'what are they up to now?'"

The Wii Bowling game allowed participants and observers to increase their daily interaction with others and to meet new people within the centres. As one participant explained, "It's expanded the socializing in this complex, and I think that was really helpful, especially for the new people."

A shy man from one of the centres had said that he would not have come and played, except that the tournament allowed him to join in. Now he has become a regular Wii bowler and still plays with the group. Another focus group participant pointed out that playing provided a reason to come together. "The only time I play Wii Bowling is when I am here because we are together. I don't have a girlfriend. I don't have a TV. There is nobody there. When we come here, we are gathering."

Stronger Social Connections. Playing the game didn't just increase the amount of interaction but created a space to build stronger connections, as one player put it "This was personal and it was neat to get to know them better." It seemed to allow players to get to know each other more and to build stronger connections. One player noted that it helped her to bond with some of the people she had known only slightly:

> It got me mixing or getting—I knew two of the girls I was playing with—I knew them quite well, but I met somebody else that I just sort of said hello to in the building. So we got together. And we've kind of bonded quite nicely and there's been people come up to watch and, you know, and you do more than just saying hello like you say in the elevator, "Hello," and that's as far as it gets. Then, they'll come up and they'll watch or they'll sort of like encourage them to kind of try it. So there's a lot of communication. I really enjoyed it.

Many participants stated that they got to know the other team members better. As one said, "We got to know our team members well, and we had a good time." Some of these bonds extended to outside the game, as mentioned by another participant: "I became better acquainted with several of the residents. And we exchanged contact information."

In the focus group, one team recapped:

> P1: We bonded.
> P2: Yes, we did. Because we were practicing together and we were there together. It was, it was wonderful.

Stronger connections were sometimes formed between people who were previously just acquaintances. As one player explained, "…when we pass each other now, we always stop and have a chat. They're different girls than I'm used to, and so it sort of added to my collection of girls (laughing)."

The playful environment fostered many of these social connections. As a participant stated, "…the fact that you mix together and have a few laughs and enjoy each other. It's good for you too, to be doing something rather than sitting in your room."

In the focus group, one participant even felt the end of the tournament, with the sudden lack of socializing, to be quite dramatic. "When it was over we felt a bit lost."

Continued Connections. Continued connections after the Wii Bowling tournament was a theme that was specific to the follow-up focus groups. Many team members remained friends and did other activities with each other. These ranged in attachment depending on the group dynamics, centre, and individual.

One woman whose team is in a seniors' community centre retold a story of ending up on a trip with one of the Wii tournament participants. Although it was not a deep relationship, it did show an increased connection.

> I did go on a trip after that with somebody that was in our group. We had a good chat on the whole trip. In fact there was a gift shop, naturally there was a gift shop but she had spent many years at Squamish and she knew about the gift shop that originated there. So she steered us to her gift shop which was a little further distance and which was much nicer. Mainly a jewellery store. It was a lovely, lovely jewellery store.

In one of the other centres, where regular activities are organized for the residents, a woman said "We exercise together. We play other games together. We played dominos yesterday." In another retirement centre, a participant stated, "Sometimes, you know, meet up at lunch time or dinner time. Share our lunch and our dinner, our bowling friends."

Some teams had much stronger connections and formed tight groups, evolving into regular social relationships in people's lives. One woman said that her group had bonded "and it's remained like that. Even [my husband] recognizes [my friend's] voice mail."

A player who had since moved out of the retirement village had formed strong connections with the ladies he bowled with, and as he expressed: "I come here and visit, what does that tell ya?"

One team seemed to form a tightly knit group that did many things together. During the tournament, they met to play and practice during morning coffee, and they were still playing at the time of the focus group. One team member said "I am not sure if it was Wii, but it did solidify a group of us." The group often went for meals, as one participant states, "More so now than before. We eat a lot more Chinese food (laughing). More cake and ice cream." They would also enter the apartment lottery together: "We seem to do that in a block too. We won about five weeks in a row and the rest of the building won't speak to us (laughing)."

Whether they formed lighter or stronger connections, many participants described how the Wii Bowling tournament helped them to better know those in their team.

5.5 Continued Play and Difficulty with New Players

The focus groups also examined whether participants continued playing Wii Bowling and whether they intended to do so in the future.

Did they Play after the Tournament? Eleven of the 14 centres reported that people there played Wii games after the tournament. Although the Wii systems were left at the centres, some participants were apparently unaware that they were there, could not figure out the set-up, or were not overly interested. One centre had a participant fall during the tournament, leaving a more negative feeling. The other centres showed differences in their Wii activities.

Many of the centres kept a regular schedule and made Wii Bowling a weekly activity. This was more frequent in assisted living centres than in independent living or community centres. Play usually took place once or twice each week. Other teams in independent living, and a few in community centres, attempted to organize weekly play on their own, but this was more difficult as it depended on individuals to organize and set up the system without a research assistant's help. As one focus group mentioned, "It would be nice if one person sort of took attendance and kept score. A team captain. Yeah, and maybe encourage others. You know." One team had difficulty with the Wii system, saying that it "took so long to get it going. It took 20–25 min."

A few teams had mini-tournaments after the large tournament. In one case two centres went to each other's buildings to compete against each other. "We've been playing against the people at the Towers. We've got that rivalry going so it's really good." The other team also commented, "We went to the manor and played the team there. Then we arranged for them to come here, but umm. G, we spoke to him and suggested that we leave it until the fall, which is more convenient for everybody. The idea is that we go there and they come here. We went once and we didn't like it." Another centre had a little tournament within their building, with four two-person teams, that lasted three weeks.

Intention to Play in the Future. Like those who played after the tournament, 11 of the groups intended to continue to play or planned to play in the future. As stated bluntly by one participant "I will as long as I'm here." Another confirmed that "we'll always play as long as we can."

However, at the time of the focus group it was the start of the summer, and many had stopped playing, with plans to start again in the fall. Participants commented that: "Everybody, I think, feels that in the fall we'll get back to our schedule. We'll all be bowling again because we like to do it." "It's a good activity to be involved in. And the management sets up everything. If they set it up for the fall we're in it." "We hope to get it going again in the fall, maybe not as well-organized but we don't have you to drive us (laughing)."

A member from a community centre who had not been able to play after the tournament suggested that, "I'll play it if there is an opportunity. I hope the government or communities can create some conditions for us to play."

"We hope to get something in house going but boy, it's people…" This final comment leads into a new theme that surfaced during the focus groups.

Difficulty with New Players. In the follow-up focus groups, some participants expressed frustration with trying to get new people involved, for a variety of reasons. Some thought that it was simply difficult to get people interested. "It was the people in the teams. Nobody else seems to want to participate." At times, this was not because they were not wanted, but rather that they seemed uninterested. As expressed by a participant:

> I just wish more people would come out to play. You know, it's nice when we have two teams. But now, we don't have that. We didn't have any audience. No people came to watch. Nobody seems to be interested here in doing things very much.

Sometimes it was somewhat related to other difficulties, as this twosome pointed out:

> P1: Or they forget what time or day it is.
> P2: We're kind of over 85.

When new players did show interest and attended one of the sessions, they sometimes found it frustrating and easily gave up. As described by one participant, "I tried recruiting people, but if they were interested they would come and try it and they would be very easily discouraged and wouldn't come the next day, or they forgot." And another stated "No, that's the trouble. We have a bit of trouble with people joining. I think they find it a little difficult, the coordination probably."

Sometimes the difficulties were due to too many people wanting to help: "We only have one problem. There was a new player and when he or she is there, everyone is telling them how to do it. Instead of just one person. It confuses them."

At the same time, some groups found new players to be frustrating and felt impatient with trying to show them how to play. "If somebody comes in and wants to learn how to play and you know, spend 5–10 min while the rest of the people are watching, you try to be patient but you think "I can set this up anytime I want and the place is open." One player suggested:

When we get new people who are not familiar with it at all and the other people are anxious to get going with it, I feel a little friction. I just have the feeling I am waiting for somebody else, when I would like to be up there bowling with the experienced people. Maybe we should have a beginners section.

One-year Follow-up Note. A year after the follow-up focus groups were done, the recreation coordinators in the centres were contacted to see how many people were still playing. Six of the 14 centres still had Wii Bowling activities. These were centres that organized the activities as part of a regular schedule. As the focus group comments hinted, those centres that required self-organization tended to fade off.

6   Discussion

In the initial Wii Bowling study, both quantitative and qualitative analysis showed an increase in socio-emotional benefits (increased social connectedness and decreased loneliness) for older adults game players. Social connectedness and loneliness often influence each other, since lacking a sense of belonging can create feelings of loneliness [33]. The initial study seemed to reinforce this idea, as both scores were affected. Even three months after, participants reflected that they had made some new connections and had stronger ties with others. It is interesting that in some cases these social connections, which were novel at first, seemed to become more familiar.

One thing to note is that social networks were to some extent already in place in the centres, as each person had some involvement through visiting, residence, or care. However, the stronger connections and increased interactions described here may have been important for building stronger positive relationships. Socio-emotional selectivity theory, as described by Carstensen [11], suggests that if relationships are often chosen by older adults for their affective quality, then environments of fun and play may be an appealing context for meeting their social connectedness needs. Gameplay may encourage a move from a simple nod in the hallway at the start of the eight weeks to stopping and chatting later on, but even this slight shift towards more familiarity may be beneficial. In this experiment, the positive affective experience of gameplay allowed for the forming of closer bonds, often seen as important for older adults' wellbeing.

Many of the connections formed by the participants in this study were related to companionship rather than support. Companionship plays an important role in meeting the social needs of older adults [26]. This is particularly important when considered together with loneliness. As seen in the qualitative findings, participants' sense of belonging increased with their more frequent interactions and as they formed stronger ties with acquaintances.

It is interesting that in the initial tournament, all players started on a relatively equal footing in terms of skill and (lack of) Wii experience. In the follow-up, however, new players had to be brought into existing, experienced groups. This was often seen as somewhat problematic because it was difficult to recruit new players, or new players had problems playing or learning the game, or the original players felt annoyed at having to help or to wait for new people to learn. There seemed to be a tension between wanting new players and the challenges of having new players, which could cause some diffi-culties for playing in the future.

Regarding difficulty in recruiting new players, it is possible that potential new recuits lacked the autonomy and competence suggested by Zonneveld & Loos [50] as needed for gameplay motivation. New players may have also felt uneasy despite desiring social contact, since feeling less than competent might create a negative emotional experience, particularly if other players felt tension. This could create an environment where newcomers might decide not to return, since they found only limited rewards at the start.

The tournament created a structured environment that motivated the players to participate. Only one group dropped out during the eight-week tournament. Although the original plan did not include support for continuing play once the intervention was completed, in some centres Wii Bowling was added to the ongoing activity schedule. Thus the tournament created an environment where people came together, and it brought them close enough to continue their newfound relationships afterwards. Digital games may be a place to create a relaxing, enjoyable environment with others in which to create new connections.

This study also confirms the importance of the role of the centre, acknowledged by Jung et al. [52]. Following our Wii Bowling tournament, play activity faded off over time when it was left to the players to organize; the centres that continued with play did so with the support of structured times and programs. For places that intend to use these systems, then, it might be useful to have specific times and to provide assistance to encourage, guide, and integrate new players.

6.1 Limitations and Future Directions

The main limitations of all phases of the study were that participants were volunteers, which often leads to attracting players who are more outgoing. Thus, it can be difficult to generalize to those who are housebound, introverted, or nervous about participating. The follow-up study also only involved a subset of the participants (just over half) who volunteered for the focus groups, and so cannot reflect the experiences of all of the tournament participants. However, at least one representative was included from each of the 20 teams.

This research could be extended by examining the changing dynamics of social relationships within groups of older adult game players. It might also be useful to create and study clubs or other ways to facilitate teams for older adults outside organizing centres. There are also many opportunities for intergenerational play that could enhance familiar social relationships, while also building new connections.

7 Conclusion

Our original Wii Bowling study provided insights into the use of digital games for increasing social connectedness and reducing loneliness among older adults. Qualitative analysis of post-tournament interviews confirmed these findings, and they were further confirmed through three-month follow-up focus groups. Many of the original participants maintained connections with some of their teammates for the three months after the study, suggesting that digital games may be useful in creating lasting social connectedness. Many centres also maintained this activity by scheduling it into their program of activities for their seniors.

Acknowledgements. We wish to thank the Social Sciences and Humanities Research Council of Canada (SSHRC) for supporting this project financially through a four-year Insight grant.

References

1. World Health Organization: Global Health and Aging (2012). http://www.who.int/ageing/publications/global_health.pdf
2. Kaufman, D.: Aging Well: Can Digital Games Help? Overview of the Project. Presented at the World Social Science Forum, Montreal, QC (2013)
3. World Health Organization: Active Aging: a Policy Framework. Geneva, World Health Organization (2002). http://whqlibdoc.who.int/hq/2002/WHO_NMH_NPH_02.8.pdf
4. McDaniel, S.A., Rozanova, J.: Canada's aging population (1986) Redux. Can. J. Aging 30(3), 511–521 (2011). doi:http://dx.doi.org.proxy.lib.sfu.ca/10.1017/S0714980811000420
5. Bowling, A., Dieppe, P.: What is successful ageing and who should define it? BMJ 331(7531), 1548–1551 (2005)
6. Phelan, E.A., Anderson, L.A., Lacroix, A.Z., Larson, E.B.: Older adults' views of "successful aging"—how do they compare with researchers' definitions? J. Am. Geratr. Soc. 52(2), 211–216 (2004)
7. Fernández-Ballesteros, R., Robine, J.M., Walker, A., Kalache, A.: Active aging: a global goal. Curr. Gerontol. Geriatr. Res. 2013(298012), 4 (2013). doi:10.1155/2013/298012
8. Forsman, A.K., Nyqvist, F., Schierenbeck, I., Gustafson, Y., Wahlbeck, K.: Structural and cognitive social capital and depression among older adults in two nordic regions. Aging Ment. Health 16(6), 771–779 (2012). doi:10.1080/13607863.2012.667784
9. Glei, D.A., Landau, D.A., Goldman, N., Chuang, Y.L., Rodríguez, G., Weinstein, M.: Participating in social activities helps preserve cognitive function: an analysis of a longitudinal, population-based study of the elderly. Int. J. Epidemiol. 34(4), 864–871 (2005). doi:10.1093/ije/dyi049
10. Theurer, K., Wister, A.: Altruistic behaviour and social capital as predictors of wellbeing among older Canadians. Ageing Soc. 30(1), 157–181 (2010). doi:http://dx.doi.org.proxy.lib.sfu.ca/10.1017/S0144686X09008848
11. Carstensen, L.L.: Motivation for social contact across the life span: a theory of socioemotional selectivity. Nebr. Symp. Motiv. 40, 209–254 (1993)
12. Park, N.S., Zimmerman, S., Kinslow, K., Shin, H.J., Roff, L.L.: Social engagement in assisted living and implications for practice. J. Appl. Gerontol. 31(2), 215–238 (2012). doi:10.1177/0733464810384480
13. Kaufman, D.: Socio-emotional benefits of digital games for older adults. In: Proceedings of the 6th International Conference on Computer Supported Education (CSEDU 2014), Barcelona, Spain. SciTePress Digital Library Online, Setubal, Portugal (2014)
14. Zhang, F., Kaufman, D.: Physical and cognitive impacts of digital games on older adults: a meta-analytic review. J Appl. Gerontol. (2015). doi:10.1177/0733464814566678
15. Astell, A.: Technology and fun for a happy old age. In: Sixsmith, A., Gutman, G. (eds.) Technologies for Active Aging. International Perspectives on Aging, vol. 9, pp. 169–187. Springer, New York (2013)

16. IJsselsteijn, W., Nap, H.H., de Kort, Y., Poels, K.: Digital game design for elderly users. In: Kapralos, B., Katchabaw, M., Rajnovich, J. (eds.) Proceedings of the 2007 Conference on Future Play, pp. 17–22. ACM, New York (2007)

17. De Schutter, B.: Never too old to play: the appeal of video games to an older audience. Games Cult. **6**(2), 155–170 (2011). doi:10.1177/1555412010364978

18. Kahlbagh, P.E., Sperandio, A.J., Carlson, A.L., Hauselt, J.: Effects of playing wii on wellbeing in the elderly: physical activity, loneliness, and mood. Activities Adapt. Aging **35**(4), 331–344 (2011). doi:10.1080/01924788.2011.625218

19. Wollersheim, D., Merkes, M., Shields, N., Liamputtong, P., Wallis, L., Reynolds, F., Koh, L.: Physical and psychosocial effects of wii video game use among older women. IJETS **8**(2), 85–98 (2010)

20. Ory, M.G., Evashwick, C.J., Glasgow, R.B., Sharkey, J.R., Browning, C.J., Thomas, S.A.: Pushing the boundaries of evidence-based research: enhancing the application and sustainability of health promotion programs in diverse populations. In: Browing, C., Thomas, S.A. (eds.) Behavioral Change: An Evidence-based Handbook for Social and Public Health, pp. 267–293. Elsevier Churchill, Edinburgh (2005)

21. Hausknecht, S., Schell, R., Zhang, F., Kaufman, D.: Building seniors' social connections and reducing loneliness through a digital game. In: Proceedings of the ICT4Ageingwell 2015, Lisbon, Portugal (2015)

22. Schell, R., Hausknecht, S., Zhang, F., Kaufman, D.: Social benefits of playing Wii Bowling for older adults. Games Cult. (in press)

23. Elder Jr., G.H.: Time, human agency, and social change: perspectives on the life course. Soc. Psychol. Q. **57**(1), 4–15 (1994)

24. Baumeister, R.F., Leary, M.R.: The need to belong: desire for interpersonal attachments as a fundamental human motivation. Psychol. Bull. **117**(3), 497–529 (1995)

25. Adams, K.B., Leibbrandt, S., Moon, H.: A critical review of the literature on social and leisure activity and wellbeing in later life. Aging Soc. **31**(4), 683–712 (2011)

26. Ashida, S., Heaney, C.A.: Differential associations of social support and social connectedness with structural features of social networks and the health status of older adults. J. Aging Health **20**(7), 872–893 (2008). doi:10.1177/0898264308324626

27. Sirven, N., Debrand, T.: Social participation and healthy ageing: an international comparison using SHARE data. Soc. Sci. Med. **67**(12), 2017–2026 (2008). doi:10.1016/j.socscimed.2008.09.056

28. Fratiglioni, L., Paillard-Borg, S., Winblad, B.: An active and socially integrated lifestyle in late life might protect against dementia. Lancet Neurol. **3**, 343–353 (2004). doi:10.1016/S1474-4422(04)00767-7

29. Cannuscio, C., Block, J., Kawachi, I.: Social capital and successful aging: the role of senior housing. Ann. Intern. Med. **139**(5 Part 2), 395–399 (2003)

30. Litwin, H., Shiovitz-Ezra, S.: Social network type and subjective wellbeing in a national sample of older Americans. Gerontologist **51**(3), 379–388 (2011). doi:10.1093/geront/gnq094

31. van Bel, D.T., Smolders, K.C.H.J., IJsselsteijn, W.A., de Kort, Y.: Social connectedness: concept and measurement. In: Callaghan, V., Kameas, A., Reyes, A., Royo, D., Weber, M. (eds.) Intelligent Environments 2009: Proceedings of the 5th International Conference on Intelligent Environments, pp. 67–74. IOS Press, Amsterdam (2009)

32. Lambert, N.M., Stillman, T.F., Hicks, J.A., Kamble, S., Baumeister, R.F., Fincham, F.D.: To belong is to matter: sense of belonging enhances meaning in life. Pers. Soc. Psychol. Bull. **39**(11), 1418–1427 (2013). doi:10.1177/0146167213499186

33. Rook, K.S.: Social relationships as a source of companionship: implications for older adults' psychological wellbeing. In: Sarason, B.R., Sarason, I.G., Gregory, R.P. (eds.) Social Support: an Interactional View, pp. 219–250. John Wiley, New York (1990)
34. Cacioppo, J.T., Patrick, W.: Loneliness: Human Nature and the Need for Social Connection. W.W. Norton & Company, New York (2008)
35. Hawkley, L.C., Cacioppo, J.T.: Loneliness matters: a theoretical and empirical review of consequences and mechanisms. Ann. Behav. Med. **40**(2), 218–227 (2010). doi:10.1007/s12160-010-9210-8
36. Pinquart, M., Sorensen, S.: Influences on loneliness in older adults: a meta-analysis. BASP **23**(4), 245–266 (2001)
37. Dykstra, P.A., van Tilburg, T.G., de Jong Gierveld, J.: Changes in older adult loneliness results from a seven-year longitudinal study. Res. Aging **27**(6), 725–747 (2005). doi:10.1177/0164027505279712
38. Buckley, C., McCarthy, G.: An exploration of social connectedness as perceived by older adults in a long-term care setting in Ireland. Geriatr. Nurs. **30**(6), 390–396 (2009). doi:10.1016/j.gerinurse.2009.09.001
39. Mannell, R.C., Kleiber, D.A.: A Social Psychology of Leisure. Venture Publishing Inc., State College, PA (1997)
40. Burnett-Wolle, S., Godbey, G.: Refining research on older adults' leisure: implications of selection, optimization, and compensation and socioemotional selectivity theories. J. Leisure Res. **39**(3), 498–513 (2007)
41. Baecker, R., Moffatt, K., Massimi, M.: Technologies for aging gracefully. Interactions **19**(3), 32–36 (2012)
42. Entertainment Software Association: Essential Facts (2015). http://www.theesa.com/wp-content/uploads/2015/04/ESA-Essential-Facts-2015.pdf
43. Entertainment Software Association (ESA) Essential Facts (2014). http://www.theesa.com/wp-content/uploads/2014/10/ESA_EF_2014.pdf
44. Delwiche, A.A., Henderson, J.J.: The players they are A-changin': the rise of older MMO gamers. J. Broadcast. Electron. Media **57**(2), 205–223 (2013). doi:10.1080/08838151.2013.787077
45. Kaufman, D., Sauvé, L., Renaud, L., Duplàa, E.: Cognitive benefits of digital games for older adults. In: Herrington, J., Viteli, J., Leikomaa, M. (eds.) Proceedings of the World Conference on Educational Media and Technology (EdMedia) 2014, pp. 289–297. Association for the Advancement of Computing in Education (AACE), Waynesville, NC (2014)
46. Nap, H.H., de Kort, Y., IJsselsteijn, W.A.: Senior gamers: preferences, motivations and needs. Gerontechnology **8**(4), 247–262 (2009)
47. Nimrod, G.: The fun culture in seniors' online communities. Gerontologist **51**(2), 226–237 (2011). doi:10.1093/geront/gnq084
48. Csikszentmihalyi, M.: Flow and education. NAMTA J. **22**(2), 2–35 (1997)
49. Sorenson, N., Pasquier, P.: The evolution of fun: automatic level design through challenge modeling. In: Ventura, D., Pease, A., Pérez y Pérez, R., Ritchie, G., Veale, T. (eds.) Proceedings of the First International Conference on Computational Creativity (ICCCX), pp. 258–267. University of Coimbra, Coimbra, Portugal (2010)
50. Zonneveld, A., Loos, E.F.: Silver gaming: ter leering ende vermaeck? [Silver Gaming: Serious Fun for Seniors?]. Tijdschr. Gerontol. Geriatr. **46**, 152–159 (2015). doi:10.1007/s12439-015-0129-1
51. Gamberini, L., Alcaniz, M., Barresi, G., Fabregat, M., Ibanez, F., Prontu, L.: Cognition, technology and games for the elderly: an introduction to the ELDERGAMES project. PsychNology **4**(3), 285–308 (2006)

52. Jung, Y., Li, K.J., Janissa, N.S., Gladys, W.L.C., Lee, K.M.: Games for a better life: effects of playing wii games on the wellbeing of seniors in a long-term care facility. In: Proceedings of the Sixth Australasian Conference on Interactive Entertainment (article 5). ACM, New York (2009)

53. Peng, W., Lin, J., Crouse, J.: Is playing exergames really exercising? a meta-analysis of energy expenditure in active video games. Cyberpsychology Behav. Soc. Netw. **14**(11), 681–688 (2011). doi:10.1089/cyber.2010.0578

54. Wiemeyer, J., Kliem, A.: Serious games in prevention and rehabilitation—a new panacea for elderly people? Eur. Rev. Aging Phys. Act. **9**(1), 41–50 (2012). doi:10.1007/s11556-011-0093-x

55. Nimrod, G.: Older adults' online communities: a qualitative analysis. Gerontologist **50**(3), 382–392 (2010)

56. Pearce, C.: The truth about baby boomer gamers – a study of over-forty computer game players. Games Cult. **3**(2), 142–174 (2008). doi:10.1177/1555412008314132

57. Russell, D.W.: UCLA loneliness scale (Version 3): reliability, validity, and factor structure. J. Pers. Assess. **66**(1), 20–40 (1996)

Surpassing Entertainment with Computer Games: Online Tools for Early Warnings of Mild Cognitive Impairment

Béla Pataki[1(✉)], Péter Hanák[2], and Gábor Csukly[3]

[1] Department of Measurement and Information Systems, Budapest University of Technology and Economics, Műegyetem rakpart 3, Budapest 1111, Hungary
pataki@mit.bme.hu
[2] Healthcare Technologies Knowledge Centre, Budapest University of Technology and Economics, Műegyetem rakpart 3, Budapest 1111, Hungary
hanak@emt.bme.hu
[3] Department of Psychiatry and Psychotherapy, Semmelweis University, Balassa utca 6, Budapest 1038, Hungary
csukly.gabor@med.semmelweis-univ.hu

Abstract. Due to population aging, *old age cognitive deficit* is becoming a mass-phenomenon. *Dementia,* its most severe variant, is *chronic, progressive, long lasting and, so far, incurable.* The early sign of a higher risk for a pathological decrease in cognition is called Mild Cognitive Impairment (MCI). Early detection of MCI is crucial for providing cost-effective care, and slowing down the deterioration. As clinical tests are infrequent and expensive, tests applicable for regular home monitoring have to be developed. In this paper, *regular but voluntary use of computer games is proposed for measuring mental changes in an entertaining way.* Basic considerations, challenges, proposed architectures, potential solutions based on virtual sensor fusion and statistical comparison of reference and test data sets, presentation of results, and proofs of the concept are described in the paper. The work was performed in the *Maintaining and Measuring Mental Wellness (M3W)* project supported by the AAL Joint Programme.

Keywords: Computer game · Silver game · Cognitive disorders · Mild cognitive impairment · MCI · Early warning · Change detection · Virtual sensor fusion · Diagnostic report · PAL test

1 Introduction

The world's population is aging: those aged 65 years or over will account for 28.7 % of the EU-28's population by 2080, compared with 18.2 % in 2013. As a result of the population movement between age groups, the EU-28's old-age dependency ratio is projected to almost double from 27.5 % in 2013 to 51.0 % by 2080 [8].

Older adults have to cope with physical and mental impairments. Old age cognitive deficit is a relatively new mass-phenomenon due to the fast growth of older populations, and the fact that dementia is chronic, progressive, long lasting and, so far, incurable. According to Alzheimer's Research UK, "the annual economic cost of dementia is

© Springer International Publishing Switzerland 2015
M. Helfert et al. (Eds.): ICT4AgeingWell 2015, CCIS 578, pp. 217–237, 2015.
DOI: 10.1007/978-3-319-27695-3_13

nearly the same as the combined economic costs of cancer and heart disease" [1]. In December 2013, the G8 dementia summit called for strengthening and joining efforts to "identify a cure or a disease-modifying therapy for dementia by 2025", and acknowledged prevention, timely diagnosis and early intervention of dementia as innovation priorities [9].

Various paper- and object-based psychological tests have been in use since the beginning of the 20th century, aiming at recognizing cognitive disorders. Recently, their computerized variants as well as neuroimaging methods have been available for diagnostic purposes in clinics. As these are expensive and need the contribution of specialists, they are not suitable for mass screening.

In this paper, we propose to use computer games for the home monitoring of eventual significant changes in mental state. This approach is advantageous as it is a regular but voluntary method. This way, more frequent assessments are possible than with the traditional clinical test scenario.

Sections 2 and 3 characterize briefly variants of cognitive impairments and their recognition possibilities. Section 4 presents the conceptual model of the proposed system for the assessment of mental changes. Section 5 describes the system developed in the Maintaining and Measuring Mental Wellness (M3W) project: first, it summarizes the so-called early pilot, then sketches the M3W ICT architecture, presents the game categories, and finally introduces the logging and scoring procedures. Section 6 discusses evaluation challenges and proposes several approaches. Section 7 overviews the diagnostic reports generated from the results of statistical evaluation. Section 8 presents proofs of the detection method. Finally, Sect. 9 summarizes our findings, and shows directions for further work.

2 Cognitive Impairments

The early sign of having a higher risk for a pathological decrease in cognition is called Mild Cognitive Impairment, abbreviated as MCI [19]; in this state, conversion to dementia is much higher (>10–15 %) than with healthy older people. The importance of recognizing the population at risk is underlined by scientific data showing that treatment initiated in the early phase can prolong this phase, and improve the ability for independence [4]. However, in the early phase of cognitive decline symptoms do not manifest clearly, and may remain unexplored for a longer period of time. Further, it is not easy to identify the stage at which the process becomes abnormal, and the affected person requires serious attention, perhaps medical intervention, as MCI is a set of symptoms rather than a specific medical condition or disease. A person with MCI has subtle problems with one or more of the following [2]:

- day-to-day memory,
- planning,
- language,
- attention,
- visuospatial skills (the ability to interpret objects and shapes).

With early detection of MCI people at risk can get advice, support and therapy in time. Early diagnosis also allows people to plan ahead while they are still able to do so. As said above, cognitive decline can be significantly slowed down in an early stage. However, early detection is rare because cognitive tests are usually performed only when there are clear signs of cognitive deficit. The natural denying effect by the older adult, their family members and friends may lead to significant additional delays.

Traditional, validated, paper-based clinical tests constitute the gold standard but they have several drawbacks. Such tests require specialist centers and highly trained professionals. Therefore, there is a growing interest in the development of computerized cognitive assessment batteries [5, 6, 15]. However, clinical tests, using either paper-based or computerized methods, are made quite infrequently, providing too sparse snapshots of the cognitive performance.

3   Gamifying MCI Detection

Regular home – remote – monitoring of changes in mental state offers a powerful alternative, even if it allows only relatively noisy and less targeted measurements. It has the advantage of frequent assessments, and thus it offers the possibility of evaluating temporal trends. Current computerized and clinically validated tests are not suitable for this purpose as they have been developed for professional use; in consequence, they are expensive, not entertaining, and require the presence of medical staff. Therefore, new measurement methodologies should be developed and validated, specifically for this strategy.

As more and more older adults use computers, and many of them play computer games regularly, this activity can be exploited for measuring their performance in those games. According to some experimental studies, this performance is related to their cognitive state. In consequence, there is a *growing interest in the development of special computer games for cognitive monitoring and training purposes,* addressing specific cognitive domains, such as verbal fluency [11], executive functions [12], or perceptual and motor functions [16].

A major challenge in using computer games instead of cognitive tests is that entertainment capability and measurement power pose contradictory requirements. There are three approaches in game development for older adults, namely

- adapting well-known, popular games (e.g., chess, Tangram or Tic-tac-toe [14], Find the Pairs, FreeCell [13]);
- transforming special clinical tests, e.g., Corsi block-tapping, paired associates learning, Wisconsin card sorting [13], into games;
- developing new games specially designed for this purpose [12].

Regular monitoring may be controlled or voluntary. Controlled monitoring works only with a highly motivated minority, the majority tends to refuse it as a possible detection of mental decline does not attract them. Further, participation in controlled monitoring endangers their preferred independence.

Our basic idea is the following: with regular but voluntary use of computer games developed or modified specifically for older adults, we may be able to measure the mental changes and tendencies over time in an entertaining way.

The problems, possible solutions and methods, presented in this paper, are based on a recent research project, Maintaining and Measuring Mental Wellness [10, 13, 17]. The ultimate goal of the project is to develop a toolset and a methodology for monitoring the mental state of older adults remotely (e.g., at home), which is a very complex task. Therefore, only the basic considerations and concepts, a few challenges, problems and solutions, the proposed architecture, and the proofs of the concept are presented in this paper. Many other important problems, such as player motivation and game selection, are not discussed here in detail.

One of the biggest challenges is to find the right balance between entertainment capability and measurement power. In order to cope with this challenge, the game set has been evolving since our early pilot experiments, performed in 2012/2013. Unfortunately, the changing of the games and the collected data poses another significant challenge as basically non-comparable data have to be compared somehow in the long run. To this end, we propose a kind of sensor-fusion approach that will be described later, in Sect. 6.

4 Conceptual Model

The basic conceptual model of the proposed system is shown in Fig. 1. The final goal is to provide appropriate long-term feedback (warning) to the user or to a caregiver, family member, medical expert, etc., when a significant change in mental state has occurred. Short-term feedback is needed as motivation to continue participation in the monitoring.

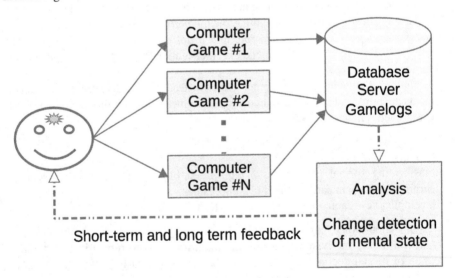

Fig. 1. Basic conceptual model of the cognitive state evaluation system.

Several games have been considered. Most of the chosen ones are logical puzzles, or games that need the intensive use of the short-term memory (its deterioration is one of the best indicators of MCI), but other important cognitive abilities and processes (attention, executive function, comprehension, language skills, planning, decision making, etc.) are targeted as well (see details in Sect. 5).

Two types of basic parameters are measured currently: the *solving time* of the puzzle, and the *amount of the good and bad steps* taken during the solution.

In Fig. 2, a typical series of performance is shown for a player playing the same game nearly 120 times. The time span of that series was 14 months. The performance is fluctuating around a mean value, and there is an outlier far from the usual values.

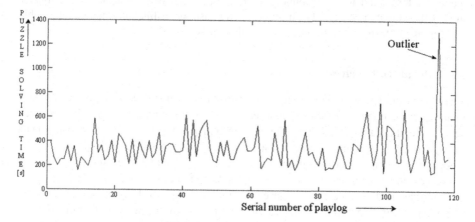

Fig. 2. Typical performance series of a player measured with a given computer game.

Beyond the general problems of such systems (e.g., data privacy concerns), this approach has its special challenges:

1. How to **measure cognitive performance** using computer games?
2. How to *cope with* the typically heavy **noise** of the uncontrolled (home) measurement environment?
3. How to **motivate people** to take part in the long run?
4. How to **compare performance** shown in different games, which is basically a special sensor-fusion problem?

After describing the ICT architecture and components in the next section, we shall propose various approaches and procedures as possible answers to these challenges.

5 ICT Architecture and Components

5.1 Early Pilot

In a one-year pilot study in 2012/2013, more than 50 volunteers registered to take part and help evaluate the framework and the games developed at that time. Due to the voluntary nature of the project only about 20 of them played regularly for nearly one year at home or in an elderly home. (Of course, the parallel development of the program package was a drawback for the players.) The average age of these regular players was 70.3, and the standard deviation was 10.9 years.

Because of the relatively short test period, its relevance was limited in regard to mental aging; nonetheless, we found some findings as clearly important for the long run as well. Parallel to the home monitoring pilot study, clinical examinations on patients with mental problems (MCI, Alzheimer's disease, etc.) were also performed [17, 18].

The software package for the early pilot was written in Java, and had to be downloaded and installed; it was a challenge in itself for many older adults. Recent advancements of internet and browser technologies have made it possible to develop the software in HTML5, JavaScript and PHP in the second phase, go online, and become available on various platforms, including touchscreen devices.

5.2   Global Architecture

The current implementation is composed of the M3W frame and the set of games – the Game Service (GS). The M3W frame ensures a unified layout and provides various services to the games, including completing and passing the gamelogs to the Data Service (DS). The Game Service can be displayed in a big-enough *iframe* in any webpage. Authentication and authorization – i.e. provision of a User Register (UR) – is the responsibility of the webserver hosting the Game Service.

For older adults, especially for those with limited computer skills and, to some extent, affected by cognitive impairment, *ease of use* (incl. easy registration and login) is *especially important*. For them, modern Single-Sign-On (SSO) solutions can be very helpful. Therefore, despite the immature status of and frequent changes in SSO applications, we have implemented such services based on an open source solution, *simpleSAMLphp* (SSP) that is used worldwide in higher education. With SSP, on the one hand, a so-called identity provider (IdP) can integrate authentication services of a number of external authentication sources, incl. social login services offered by social network providers, such as Google, Facebook and LinkedIn. On the other hand, a webservice can be amended by a so-called service provider (SP) with SSP such that this webservice can utilize the authentication mechanisms of one or more IdPs.

In the simplest case, User Register (UR), Game Service (GS) and Data Service (DS) can run on the same server (e.g., a Drupal 7 instance may be used for this purpose). A simple distributed architecture is depicted in Fig. 3.

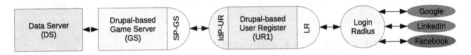

Fig. 3. Simple distributed architecture.

Sometimes more sophisticated architectures are needed. For example, with a high number of users the load on a single GS may be too high, and a second GS has to be added.

In another situation, privacy concerns or regulations might require that the UR remain under the authority of an institution, or within a country, so the UR must be duplicated or even multiplied. Further, the collected data might be considered as sensitive despite that they contain no personal data only an integer player identifier. In such situations, it must be ensured that the DS be duplicated or multiplied. SSP ensures the necessary scalability and connectivity also in such cases. Figure 4 illustrates a situation where a complex M3W system is realized by two DS, three GS, three UR and six SSP instances, and other external services.

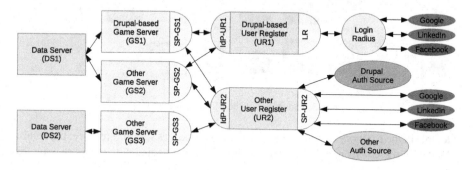

Fig. 4. Complex distributed architecture.

Note that both GS and UR services can be realized without Drupal.

5.3 Cognitive Abilities and Game Categories

Cognitive abilities are mental skills needed to carry out tasks. They are mechanisms of how we learn, remember, plan, execute, solve problems, pay attention, etc. Major categories of cognitive abilities are perception, attention, memory, motor skills, language skills, visual and spatial processing, and executive functions.

Cognitive tests – traditional or computerized – are designed to measure one of these abilities in order to maximize their assessment capability; they are not designed for frequent use. However, *in case of cognitive games,* their *measurement potential must be accompanied by entertaining power* as they must motivate the user to play regularly for a long time.

The M3W set of games tries to satisfy both major requirements. Each game belongs to at least one of five cognitive categories: attention, executive function, language skill, memory, and visuospatial skill (see Fig. 5).

Most games try to focus on one cognitive category; e.g., *Birds, Boxes, Differences* or *Jigsaw Puzzle* deal with attention; *Find the Pairs* (known also as *Memory Game)* with memory; *Letters* and *Guess Words* with language skills. Games belonging to the category executive function are usually more complex, i.e. more demanding; examples for such games are *FreeCell, Sudoku, Blocks, Pipes, Masyu,* or *Labyrinth* (because of its complexity the latter was added for entertainment rather than assessment).

Additionally, a few known psychological tests – so far, the PAL test and gamified versions of the Corsi block tapping test and the Wiconsin card test – are also made

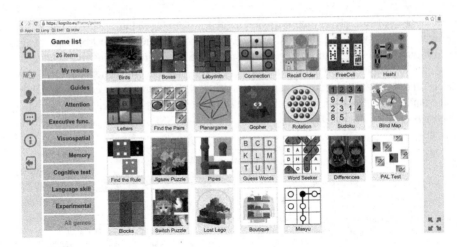

Fig. 5. Snapshot of the M3W playground.

available in the category cognitive test. They may be used as sort of reference: the results gained with these tests may be compared with the results gained with the more complex games.

5.4 Game Logging

As mentioned in Sect. 4, the solving time and the amount of good and bad steps have recently been used for statistical analysis. However, parameters describing the game settings, the gaming platform and the course of playing the game are also recorded in the game logs; these data can and will be used later to compute suitable indicators.

Settings are game-specific such as difficulty level, word length and language, turning or moving speed, appearance time, board size, etc. *Platform parameters* include monitor resolution, browser version, operating system, the use of mouse, touchpad or touchscreen, etc. The *course of playing the game* is described by all significant mouse clicks or touches; they are logged with timestamps. (The analysis of the actual path of the cursor would provide important information about the player, but it will be investigated in the future. Currently only the events, e.g. mouse clicks are analyzed.)

Game logs are *json-objects,* saved into files. Each game log consists of five components and several subcomponents:

1. Game descriptor (numeric identifier, name, category, version).
2. Player identifier (numeric identifier).
3. Parameters (date, settings and other options, seed of psuedo-random number generator, platform, game log version).
4. Events (game-specific series of time-stamped event-items).
5. Statistics (score, play time, game-specific aggregated values).

5.5 Score Calculation

Various faults may lead to score deductions such as long playtimes, bad moves, wrong mouse clicks, erroneous selections, etc. Although the score calculation method is common, *fault types* vary from game to game. A *threshold,* a *limit* and a *weight* is assigned to each fault type in every game.

- *Fault value:* it is the measure of the extent or seriousness of an actual fault.
- *Threshold:* if the fault value does not exceed its threshold the error component is zero.
- *Limit:* it determines the effect of the fault value on the *combined error:* limits closer to the threshold yield bigger effects on the combined error. In other words, limit determines the *slope* of the *score calculation curves* in Fig. 7.
- *Weight:* it also determines the effect of the fault value – in comparison to other fault values – on the combined error. Smaller weights have smaller effects.

From the fault value and the corresponding threshold, limit and weight values an *error component* is calculated. Figure 6 illustrates the calculation of an error component where threshold, limit and weight are the same for a given fault type while the fault value varies. Note that only fault values exceeding their thresholds lead to score deductions.

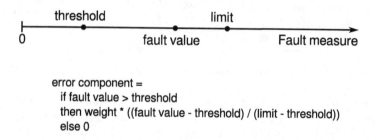

error component =
if fault value > threshold
then weight * ((fault value - threshold) / (limit - threshold))
else 0

Fig. 6. Error component calculation.

Error components are computed and summed up by the score calculator to result the combined error. This is then used to determine the score deduction, and produce the final score (see Fig. 7).

The common score calculator has four formal parameters: *currentValues* (aka fault values), *goodValues* (aka thresholds), *acceptableValues* (aka limits) and *weights.* All formal parameters are *n-tuples,* having the same number of elements. The ith element of an *n-tuple* is related to the ith elements of the other *n-tuples.* One element of the *n-tuple* passed as *currentValues* to the score calculator corresponds to one fault.

For example, if excess play time and bad moves produce faults in a game, then a 2-tuple is passed where the first element corresponds to the excess play time, and the second element to the bad moves.

Scoring follows the same principle and procedure for every game. The highest reachable score depends on the difficulty settings. (The actual difficulty level is chosen by the player from a predefined set of possibilities in the game settings menu.) On the lowest and highest difficulty levels the maximal score is 600 and 1000, respectively.

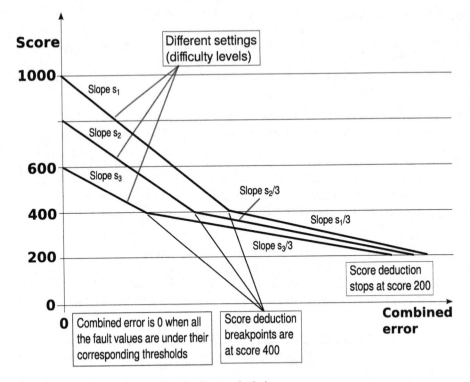

Fig. 7. Score calculation curves.

High score limits on intermediate difficulty levels (i.e., between the lowest and highest levels) are distributed linearly (see Fig. 7). With a single difficulty level, the maximal score is 1000. With two difficulty levels, the maximal scores are 600 and 1000; with three difficulty levels, 600, 800 and 1000, etc.

When the final score decreases to 400, further deductions are reduced to one-third of their original values. When the final score reaches 200, score deduction stops. Both rules were introduced to motivate the poorly performing players.

As an example, let us assume that

- there are three difficulty levels in a game;
- there are two fault values: play time and number of bad moves;
- parameter values for the play time: threshold = 20 s, limit = 100 s, weight = 0.6, fault value = 30 s;
- parameter values for the number of bad moves: threshold = 10, limit = 50, weight = 0.4, fault value = 30;
- the lowest difficulty level is chosen.

The score computation takes into account that

1. score maximum is 600 on the lowest level;
2. both fault values (of the play time and the number of bad moves) are above their thresholds;

3. for the play time, the error component is $0.6*(30-20)/(100-20) = 3/40$;
4. for the number of bad moves, the error component is $0.4*(30-10)/(50-10) = 8/40$;
5. the combined error is $3/40 + 8/40 = 11/40$;
6. the *score deduction basis* is the score maximum on the current level (600 in this example) minus 200 (the value where the score deduction stops); now its value is 400;
7. the score value is rounded to the nearest integer.

The actual score deduction in this example is $400*(11/40) = 110$, and thus the final score is $600-110 = 490$.

If the actual score deduction were more than $600-400 = 200$, then the deduction would be calculated in two steps. For example, a deduction of 300 would result in a deduction of $200 + 100/3 = 233.3$, rounded to 233. Therefore, the score would be $600-233 = 367$ points in this case.

Correct score calculation is a crucial issue that needs regular refinement since it is used for change detection as well as motivation. Fine tuning is possible by properly selecting values for thresholds, limits and weights.

Primary score calculation is performed by the games themselves. The primary score is the basis for the immediate feedback to the user (see Fig. 8).

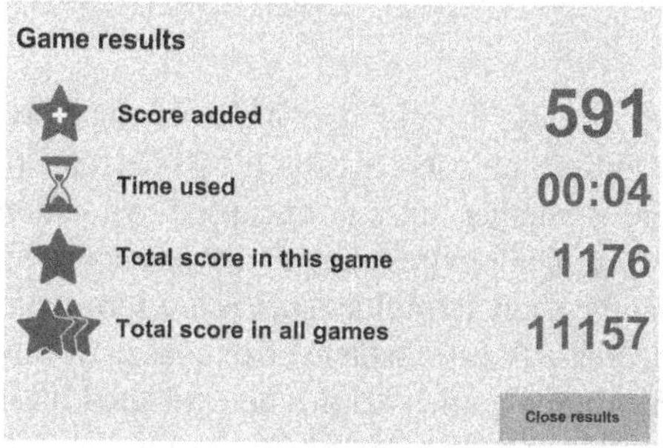

Game results

☆	Score added	**591**
⧗	Time used	**00:04**
★	Total score in this game	1176
★★★	Total score in all games	11157

Close results

Fig. 8. Snapshot of a game result.

Since all original game logs are stored, score calculation may be refined later in order to improve our assessment methods, and thus the recognition of changes in mental wellness. Secondary score calculation is performed when stored game logs are reprocessed and uploaded into the database. The secondary score is used as an indicator of cognitive performance. More sophisticated indicators might also be computed.

6   Suggestions to Meet the Challenges

To assess the cognitive state, it is assumed that performance measured in playing computer games correlates with cognitive wellness. As it will be shown in Sect. 8, there is indirect evidence that this assumption is valid.

The measurement of the mental state on an absolute scale is very difficult as it depends on education, physical health, etc. For our purpose, fortunately, it is enough to detect only **the change** in a person's cognitive performance, and it is an easier task. For measuring change, a *reference is needed*. There are two possibilities: the performance of a person can be compared to the *performance of other persons in a reference group;* or it can be compared to a *previously measured reference of the same person.*

Because the person-to-person comparison is affected by several parameters that are unknown with this voluntary, uncontrolled method (education, physical abilities, family conditions, profession, environment, etc.) the comparison to the same person's previous performance was chosen (c.f. Fig. 9).

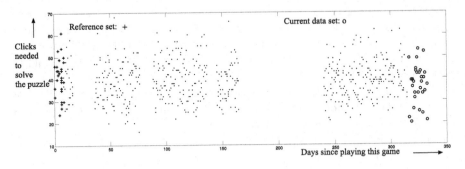

Fig. 9. Performance measure of a player during nearly one year.

To cope with the heavy noise present, data are cleaned before analysis: outliers are detected and omitted. Outliers are usually caused by interrupts (due to social or physiological reasons). There is another noise term caused by random differences between consecutive puzzles, by minor environmental disturbances, by tiredness, etc. It is reasonably assumed that the short-term fluctuations are zero-mean, stable, independent random variables. To decrease the assessment error caused by this noise term, performance measured only in a single game will not be evaluated; in its stead, performance measured on a reference set will be compared to performance on the current set (c.f. Fig. 9).

While our goal is to detect the decline of performance, in some periods improvements can occur as well. The assumption is that the decline is preceded by a longer period where the situation is stable, or deteriorating very slowly. Therefore, the reference is chosen as the group of consecutive games in which the person has shown stable performance (see Figs. 9 and 16).

The puzzle difficulty and the short-term change of cognitive performance are both zero mean random variables. The very slow, long-term change of the cognitive state is modeled differently. Therefore, if a change is detected in one of the integral characteristics (mean, median, standard deviation), or generally in the distribution of the composite random variable (mental state plus game noise), then it is caused by the slowly changing component modeling the mental state.

In Fig. 10, the distributions of the same performance measure (puzzle solving time) in the same game are shown for two players. In each diagram two performance distributions of the given player are drawn (dotted lines: distributions of reference data, solid lines: distributions of current data). Of course, the performance distributions of the same

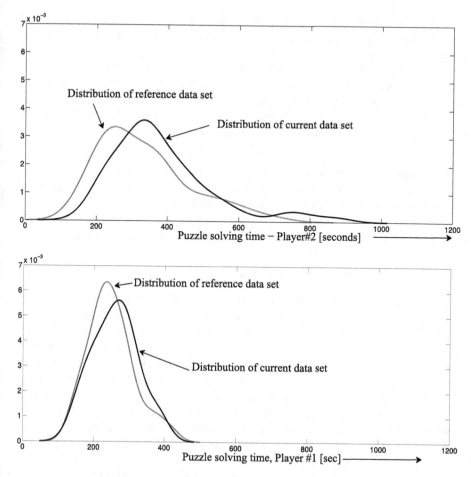

Fig. 10. Performance measure distributions of two players.

players in two time periods will not be exactly the same, but statistically the identical distribution assumption cannot be rejected. However, for different players, not only the parameters of the distributions differ from player to player but the shapes are different as well.

It was investigated whether the parameter distributions are Gaussian ones or not. The Lilliefors test rejected the normality hypothesis in most of the cases. Therefore, nonparametric tests are suggested to check if the distribution has changed or not.

6.1 Nonparametric Tests

There are several applicable nonparametric tests, for example the Mann-Whitney U test, the Kolmogorov-Smirnov two-sample test, or the Wilcoxon signed-rank test.

Any of these nonparametric test methods can be used to compare the distribution of the reference subset with the distribution of the currently examined subset of the time series, and normality is not necessary.

If we detect a difference between the distributions of the two sub-samples, and the current part of the series has a smaller average (of ranks, of scores, etc.), then the player shows performance degradation. Up to now, the Kolmogorov-Smirnov two-sample test and the chi-square test were extensively used. It will be investigated later which one is the optimal statistical hypothesis test for this kind of problems.

The following findings were obtained:

- The results, gained with the Kolmogorov-Smirnov two-sample test and the chi-square test, have confirmed that both the stability and the change in the parameters are reliably estimated with these statistical hypothesis tests.
- In case of a new game a learning phase occurs when results are improving. The reference is meaningful only when the performance is stabilized (c.f. Fig. 16).

6.2 Sensor Fusion with Games as Sensors

Motivation of older adults to play frequently and regularly with the computer games is one of the most important challenges to solve. Early detection is the purpose; but the main problem is that nobody knows when the abnormal change will happen; maybe only after many years, or in some persons' life never. Therefore, the motivation must be kept alive probably for years. It is a very complex problem itself; so only some aspects are discussed here. A basic assumption is that although there is an intrinsic motivation that everybody wants to sustain mental abilities and an independent life of good quality, generally it is not enough as a motivation in the long-run. There must be other, extrinsic motivations too, e.g., entertaining ways of measurement, and short-term, immediate feedback (c.f. Figs. 1 and 8), encouraging the user to play further (e.g., scores, symbolic rewards, encouraging messages).

Unfortunately, most people do not enjoy playing the same game for years. Therefore, in different time periods different games will be played by the same person. In order to preserve the level of motivation of the players, various games are offered (c.f. Figs. 1 and 5). – In addition, as mentioned earlier, reprogrammed or improved games and more sophisticated logging may replace older ones as assessment methods are improving while time passes by, or technology changes occur. – The performance indicators measured with different games should somehow be compared to each other. This implies a sensor fusion and estimation problem; this was discussed in our previous paper [3].

In Fig. 11, the sensor fusion scenario is illustrated. Architecturally, the scenario is a usual sensor fusion arrangement where computer games are the sensors. The most important difference is that in a usual sensor fusion arrangement the sampling is regular, typically periodic, and the sensors are sampling parallel in the same time instant. In the computer game fusion scenario only one game (sensor) is used in a time instant, and the sampling intervals are irregular. Therefore, the currently *suggested* method is to *normalize all the performance results and combine them in time.*

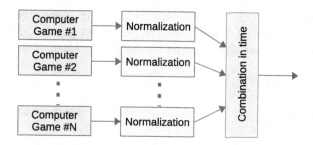

Fig. 11. The sensor fusion architecture.

We are using *a rough quantization* based on *the reference set's distribution.* Only *5 levels* are used (typically non equidistant levels), and *the quantization thresholds* are defined such that *the reference set will have uniform distribution.* (Approximately the same number of data will be at each level.) In that case, *only the uniformity of the current data has to be checked.* The method is illustrated in Fig. 12. In the future, the possibility of applying other fusion methods will be investigated.

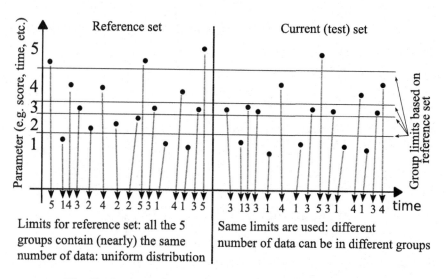

Fig. 12. Reference set based quantization used for normalization.

This quantization process results in a time series of group labels (1, 2, 3, 4, 5) which is independent of the game used. If the performance is improving then the distribution of the current (test) set will not be uniform, more 4 and 5 labels will be in the set than 1 and 2 labels. If the current performance is worse than the reference one, the 1 and 2 labels will dominate the test set. Because this procedure produces a label set which is independent of the actual game, the results of different games can be combined easily. It results in a current (test) label set of several games that are close to each other in time.

In Fig. 9, another effect is clearly present: there are gaps in the playing activity due to health problems or social reasons. Analysis of the data gaps has shown that a few week long interrupts do not change the performance significantly.

7   Diagnostic Reports

Currently, there are two basic types of diagnostic reports: reports on changes of mental conditions, and reports on specific test results.

7.1   Report on Mental Condition Changes

As mentioned above, data collected by the tests and games undergo extensive post-processing, including statistical evaluation. The aim of statistical evaluation is to detect significant changes in a player's cognitive performance.

Figure 13 illustrates the results of a statistical analysis.

M3W Trend Report

Demo version. Player id: ▆▆.

Game set	Reference sample time span	Test sample time span	Reference distribution	Test distribution	P-value	Change
(130)	2014-09-14 18:18:27 / 2014-10-23 16:56:35	2014-11-23 08:00:23 / 2015-01-29 22:14:51	[8, 9, 8, 9, 9]	[11, 8, 2, 10, 9]	0.3950	
(130)	2014-09-14 18:18:27 / 2014-10-28 13:01:27	2014-12-02 18:29:22 / 2015-01-30 23:01:33	[9, 9, 9, 9, 9]	[17, 3, 3, 8, 9]	0.0827	
(130)	2014-09-14 18:18:27 / 2014-10-28 13:01:27	2014-12-02 18:56:40 / 2015-02-02 12:48:35	[9, 9, 9, 9, 9]	[16, 3, 3, 8, 10]	0.0990	
(190)	2014-09-12 20:39:48 / 2014-10-25 22:31:28	2015-03-23 22:44:50 / 2015-04-12 04:45:43	[8, 10, 10, 10, 12]	[2, 12, 2, 1, 0]	0.0028	–
(190)	2014-09-12 20:39:48 / 2014-10-25 22:31:28	2015-03-25 15:40:36 / 2015-04-15 18:45:27	[8, 10, 10, 10, 12]	[2, 9, 2, 1, 0]	0.0185	–
(190)	2014-09-12 20:39:48 / 2014-10-25 22:31:28	2015-03-28 17:54:18 / 2015-04-16 10:50:04	[8, 10, 10, 10, 12]	[2, 7, 2, 0, 0]	0.0261	–
(190)	2014-09-12 20:39:48 / 2014-10-25 22:31:28	2015-03-30 16:03:45 / 2015-04-22 23:45:49	[8, 10, 10, 10, 12]	[2, 5, 1, 0, 0]	0.0646	
(190)	2014-09-12 20:39:48 / 2014-10-25 22:31:28	2015-03-30 16:04:52 / 2015-04-26 16:50:52	[8, 10, 10, 10, 12]	[1, 3, 0, 0, 0]	0.1165	
(190)	2014-09-12 20:39:48 / 2014-10-25 22:31:28	2015-03-31 12:42:43 / 2015-04-28 18:03:05	[8, 10, 10, 10, 12]	[1, 1, 0, 0, 0]	0.4959	
(290)	2014-09-14 17:26:47 / 2014-10-21 08:18:56	2014-11-20 17:42:45 / 2015-01-18 11:31:09	[7, 7, 7, 7, 8]	[2, 5, 13, 4, 16]	0.0842	
(290)	2014-09-14 17:26:47 / 2014-10-23 16:13:22	2014-11-24 13:19:45 / 2015-01-19 13:21:47	[8, 8, 8, 8, 9]	[2, 5, 12, 3, 18]	0.0349	+
(290)	2014-09-14 17:26:47 / 2014-10-23 16:13:22	2014-11-27 14:40:46 / 2015-01-20 09:58:09	[8, 8, 8, 8, 9]	[2, 5, 11, 3, 19]	0.0315	+
(290)	2014-09-14 17:26:47 / 2014-10-23 16:13:22	2014-11-28 09:24:15 / 2015-01-21 09:18:37	[8, 8, 8, 8, 9]	[2, 3, 10, 3, 22]	0.0079	+

Fig. 13. Excerpts from a diagnostic trend report on mental condition changes.

Change detection, as explained in other parts of this paper, is based on comparing a test sample against a reference sample for a bunch of games. If a test sample shows improvement in cognitive performance (e.g. during the early learning phase with a game) then this test sample will be used later as the new reference sample, otherwise the old reference sample is kept.

In Fig. 13, the following columns are shown:

Game Set: identifiers of those games whose results are combined in the sample.
Test Sample Time Span: first and last date of the data in the test sample.
Reference Sample Time Span: first and last date of the data in the reference sample.
Test Distribution: amount of data at the 5 quantization levels characterizing the distribution of the test sample.
Reference Distribution: amount of data at the 5 quantization levels characterizing the distribution of the reference sample.
P-value: probability of the conclusion.
Change: + *(plus)* means improvement; - *(minus)* means deterioration; *empty cell* means no significant change.

7.2   Report on PAL Test Results

Figure 14 shows a diagnostic report that is generated from the measurement data collected by performing the PAL test; the parameters are either measured, or computed.

M3W Diagnostic Report

Demo version for PAL test

Full name:		Birth name:	
Birth year:		Social security id:	
User name:		Player id:	
Email address:			

Day and time:	2015-08-03 07:12:57	Playtime (s):	527

Parameter	Outcome	Low limit	High limit
Count of total errors	12	0	73
Count of total errors with 1 shape, stages 1 and 2	0	0	19
Count of total errors with 2 shapes, stages 3 and 3	0	0	19
Count of total errors with 3 shapes, stages 5 and 6	0	0	19
Count of total errors with 6 shapes, stage 7	2	0	10
Count of total errors with 8 shapes, stage 8	10	0	10
Count of total errors, adjusted	12	0	73
Count of total errors with 1 shape, adjusted	0	0	19
Count of total errors with 2 shapes, adjusted	0	0	19
Count of total errors with 3 shapes, adjusted	0	0	19
Count of total errors with 6 shapes, adjusted	2	0	10
Count of total errors with 8 shapes, adjusted	10	0	10
Mean count of errors to success	1.5	0	10.0
Mean count of trials to success	1.375	0	5.0
Count of total trials	11	0	50
Count of total trials (adjusted)	11	0	50
Memory score on first trial	14	0	26
Number of stages completed	8	0	8
Number of stages completed on first trial	6	0	8

Fig. 14. Diagnostic report example with PAL Test results.

According to various scientific examinations the Paired Associates Learning (PAL) test discriminates well healthy subjects from subjects living with MCI (see Sect. 8).

Therefore, psychiatrists – our partners in the M3W project – started to use the M3W version of the PAL test as an auxiliary diagnostic tool.

Low and high limit values will possibly change as we collect more diagnostic experiences with the PAL Test.

Similar diagnostic reports can be generated from the results of other tests and games. Of course, further work is needed to refine such reports, and adjust them to the needs of the practicing psychiatrists.

8   Proof of the Concept

Due to the long time needed to detect a critical cognitive change, no direct proof could be collected during the project till now. Nonetheless, by *analyzing the game logs* – more than *150 voluntary persons produced over 400 thousand game logs* by playing the games during the second pilot; both the number of regular players and the amount of game logs have tripled during the last six months which shows clearly that older persons are interested in mental training with the help of computer games – some *important facts* can be shown.

To provide some calibration, one of the computerized cognitive tests (Paired Associates Learning, PAL) was implemented in the M3W project, and players were asked to perform it. Studies have shown that MCI patients performed poorly on this test [7]. Analyzing the performance of the voluntary players, it turned out that their performance shown in the computer games correlates to their performance measured by the PAL test [17, 18].

In the PAL test, cards turn up in random positions after each other for 3 s, with abstract shapes shown on one or more cards. Other cards remain blank depending on the difficulty level. When all the shapes have been shown, the previously shown shapes appear one by one in the center of the play area, and the player has to choose the card where that shape has appeared earlier. The test consists of five different levels in eight stages in total, while the number of the shapes increases from 1 to 8 on the different stages. The player has 10 trials to complete a given stage, otherwise the test ends. The arrangement of the cards is asymmetric in the test, and it changes from stage to stage.

In Fig. 15, *PAL test performance versus average puzzle solving time of four players is shown.*

The PAL test was characterized by the trials needed to reach the highest level performed by the given player. Although there were much more participants who performed PAL tests, these 4 players were selected for demonstration as they all played more than 90 FreeCell games. The outliers were omitted, and the averages of the playtimes were taken.

In a current study [18] brain magnetic resonance (MR) examination was performed on 34 healthy older adults. Beyond the MR examination, paper based and computerized neuropsychological tests (i.e., PAL test) and computer games were applied. There was a correlation between the number of attempts and the time required to complete the Find the Pairs game and the volume of the entorhinal cortex, the temporal pole, and the hippocampus. There was also a correlation between the results of the PAL test and the Find the Pairs game.

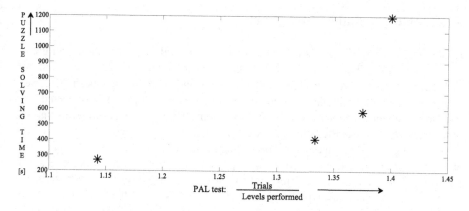

Fig. 15. Performance reached at PAL tests vs puzzle solving time in one of the games.

Although no *healthy → MCI* transition occurred during the research period, the other change: significant improvement was detected several times. In Fig. 16, performance of a player learning a new game is shown.

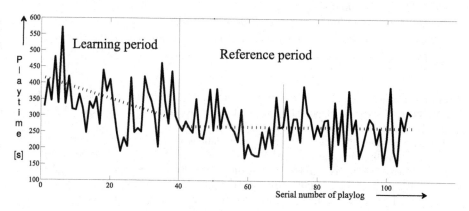

Fig. 16. Performance of a player learning a new game.

With the Kolmogorov-Smirnov (KS) two-sample test our *null hypothesis* is that *the distributions are the same.* In the situation illustrated by Fig. 16 this null hypothesis is

- *rejected* when the learning period is compared to the reference period since the KS two-sample test results $p = 0.0005$, well below the typical threshold value of $p = 0.05$;
- *accepted* when the first and second halves of the reference period are compared since the KS two-sample test results $p = 0.28$, well above the typical threshold value of $p = 0.05$.

9 Conclusion and Future Work

Home monitoring of possible significant changes in mental state using computer games has been proposed. This approach is advantageous because it is a regular but voluntary method. Some of the problems have been analyzed, and solutions have been suggested. The system assumes voluntary participation; therefore, various games have been developed to sustain motivation in the long run. In the game battery there are both well-known, popular games and modified clinical tests; it is continuously evolving.

For change detection in cognitive performance the comparison of actual data against historical data gained from the very same person is proposed, i.e. a reference set of performance results are to be compared to the current set of results using statistical hypothesis tests. The null hypothesis is that the two sets are of the same distribution. Until the null-hypothesis cannot be rejected, the stability of the mental state can be assumed.

In the future,

- *further pilots have to be launched to validate the method by more clinical tests;*
- *the most appropriate games for both entertainment and measurement purposes should be further investigated;*
- *the feasibility of multiplayer games is to be analyzed;*
- *collected but currently not analyzed data should be involved into the examinations;*
- *the potential in the evaluation of the failed games should be investigated.*

Acknowledgements. This research was performed in the Maintaining and Measuring Mental Wellness (M3W) project, supported by the AAL Joint Programme (ref. no. AAL-2009-2-109) and the Hungarian KTIA (grant no. AAL_08-1-2011-0005).

The authors gratefully acknowledge the contributions of their project partners in Greece, Luxembourg, Switzerland and Hungary. We would like to express our special thanks to (1) E. Sirály, Semmelweis University, for her contribution to the clinical examinations with real patients using the PAL test and a selection of the M3W games; (2) N. Kiss and Á. Póczik, Budapest University of Technology and Economics, for the improvement and unification of the logging and scoring procedures; (3) L. Ketskeméty, Budapest University of Technology and Economics, for exploring and elaborating various statistical evaluation algorithms.

References

1. Alzheimer's Society, UK, Dementia statistics (2014). http://www.alzheimersresearchuk.org/dementia-statistics/. Accessed April 2015
2. Alzheimer's Society, Mild Cognitive Impairment (2015). http://www.alzheimers.org.uksite/scripts/documents_info.php?documentID=120. Accessed April 2015
3. Breuer, P., Csukly, G., Hanák, P., Ketskeméty, L., Pataki, B.: Home monitoring of mental state with computer games. In: ACHI 2015 8th International Conference on Advances in Computer-Human Interactions (2015)
4. Budd, D., et al.: Impact of early intervention and disease modification in patients with predementia Alzheimer's disease: a Markov model simulation. Clinicoecon Outcomes Res. **3**, 189–195 (2011)

5. Cantab test battery, Cambridge Cognition (2015). http://www.cambridgecognition.com/. Accessed April 2015

6. Dwolatzky, T.: The mindstreams computerized assessment battery for cognitive impairment and dementia. In: PETRA 2011, May 2011, pp. 501–504 (2011). ISBN: 978-1-4503-0772-7

7. Égerházi, A., Berecz, R., Bartók, E., Degrell, I.: Automated neuropsychological test battery (CANTAB) in mild cognitive impairment and in Alzheimer's disease. Prog. Neuro-Psychopharmacol. Biol. Psychiatry **31**, 746–751 (2007)

8. Eurostat, Population structure and ageing (2014). http://ec.europa.eu/eurostat/statistics-explained/index.php/Population_structure_and_ageing. Accessed April 2015

9. Gov.UK, G8 dementia summit agreements (2013). https://www.gov.uk/government/publications/g8-dementia-summit-agreements. Accessed March 2015

10. Hanák, P., et al.: Maintaining and measuring mental wellness. In: Proceedings of the XXVI. Neumann Kollokvium, November 2013, pp. 107–110 (2013) (in Hungarian)

11. Jimison, H., Pavel, M. Le, T.: Home-based cognitive monitoring using embedded measures of verbal fluency in a computer word game. In: 30th Annual International IEEE EMBS Conference, August 2008, pp. 3312–3315 (2008). doi:10.1109/IEMBS.2008.4649913

12. López-Martínez, A., et al.: Game of gifts purchase: computer-based training of executive functions for the elderly. In: IEEE 1st International Conference on Serious Games and Applications for Health (SeGAH), November 2011, pp. 1–8 (2011), Print ISBN: 978-1-4673-0433-7 doi:10.1109/SeGAH.2011.6165448

13. M3W Maintaining and Measuring Mental Wellness (2015). AAL Joint Programme project (ref. no. AAL-2009-2-109) https://m3w-project.eu/. Accessed April 2015

14. Menza-Kubo, V., Morán, A.L.: UCSA: a design framework for usable cognitive system for the worried-well. Pers. Ubiquitous Comput. **17**(6), 1135–1145 (2013). ISSN:1617-4909. doi:10.1007/s00779-012-0554-x

15. MindStreams (2015). http://www.mind-streams.com/. Accessed April 2015

16. Ogomori, K., Nagamachi, M., Ishihara, K., Ishihara, S., Kohchi, M.: Requirements for a cognitive training game for elderly or disabled people. In: International Conference on Biometrics and Kansai Engineering, September 2011, pp 150–154 (2011). E-ISBN 978-0-7695-4512-7, Print-ISBN 978-1-4577-1356-9, doi:10.1109/ICBAKE.2011.30

17. Sirály, E., et al.: Differentiation between mild cognitive impairment and healthy elderly population using neuropsychological tests. Neuropsychopharmacol. Hung. **15**(3), 139–146 (2013)

18. Sirály, E., et al.: Monitoring the early signs of cognitive decline in elderly by computer games: an MRI study. PLoS ONE **10**(2), e0117918 (2015). doi:10.1371/journal.pone.0117918

19. Werner, P., Korczyn, A.D.: Mild cognitive impairment: Conceptual, assessment, ethical, and social issues. Clin. Interv. Aging **3**(3), 413–420 (2008)

Author Index

States